pig•ging out \ ,pig-ing 'aut \ *vb*. **1**: to consume large quantities of food with or without guilt **2**: eating as much as you want of what you want when you want **3**: the reason for living **syn** see GORGING, PORKING, SCARFING

THE JOY OF PIGGING OUT

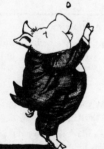

DAVID HOFFMAN

with original illustrations by
Jim Jinkins and Howard Hoffman

WARNER BOOKS

A Warner Communications Company

Copyright © 1983 by David Hoffman
All rights reserved.
Warner Books, Inc., 666 Fifth Avenue, New York, NY 10103

(w) A Warner Communications Company

Printed in the United States of America

First printing: November 1983
10   9   8   7   6   5

Illustrations by Jim Jinkins and Howard Hoffman
Cover design by Jim Jinkins
Book design by Giorgetta Bell McRee

LIBRARY OF CONGRESS CATALOGING IN PUBLICATION DATA

Hoffman, David, 1953–
The joy of pigging out.

Includes indexes.
1. Food habits—United States.   2. Restaurants,
lunch rooms, etc.—United States—Directories.
3. Grocery trade—United States—Dictionaries.   I. Title
II. Title: Pigging Out.
TX357.H58   1983   641'.01'3   83-14808
ISBN 0-446- 37958-1

THANKS to . . .

. . . the numerous professionals, businesses, public relations firms, trade organizations, and metro magazine editorial staffs who provided information integral to the compilation of this book—particularly Houston restaurant critic Jo Ann Horton, Jan Visser (*Chicago*), Gail Friedman (*Washingtonian*), Linda Matys (*New Orleans*), and Gwendelyn Korney (*San Francisco*)—and Warner Books sales reps Barrett Hargreaves, Alan Nussbaum, Jill Serio, and Woodrow Tracy.

. . . three without whom this book really *would* have been impossible: Leah Komaiko, for saying, "You should meet my friend Annie"; Annie Brody, for saying, "Work up a proposal and I'll try to sell it"; and Patti Breitman, for having the good sense to say, "I want it."

. . . those (now a few pounds heavier or, at the very least, strict vegetarians) who supplied recommendations, suggestions, or appetites: Holley and Bob Agulnek, Lisa Allen, Judi Cipnick and John Casey, Cathie Collier, Debby Cohen, Donna Forman, Bob Hattoy, Daamen Krall, Burt Levitch, Brian Levy, Harriet Lipkin, Mollie MacDonald, Terry Moore and Janet Lampe, Wanda Parton and Michael Bobenko, Susan Reins, Debbie Sabel, Steve Schatzberg, Lisa and Richard Trachtman, Lynn and John Tuck, Sally Vitsky, David Weinstein; and those who endlessly supplied all three: Andrea Marquit, Jan and Harold Pomerantz, and especially Leslie Zerg.*

. . . Mothers, other than my own, whose refrigerators I have known and loved: Eva Cohen (Los Angeles), Gloria Marquit (Brooklyn), and Catherine Moore (St. Louis).

. . . Mom, Dad, Susie, Chris, and Howard . . . for the obvious.

*Above and beyond the call of duty.

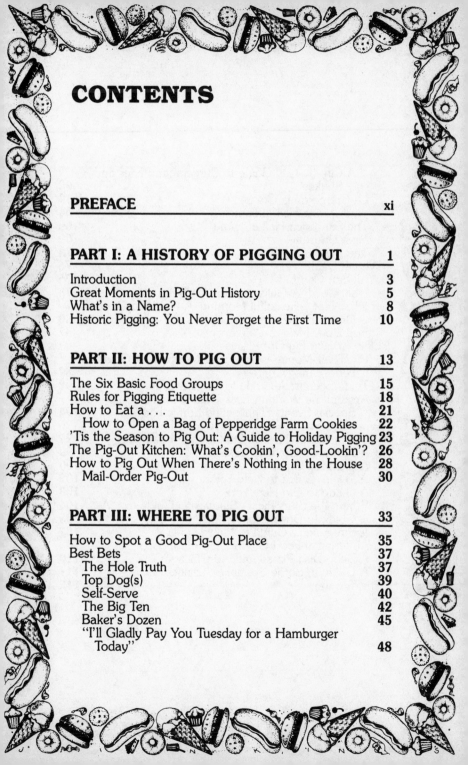

CONTENTS

PREFACE

The warning signs are unmistakable: the longing stare, the sweaty palms, the butterflies in the stomach, the rapid rate of the heart.

Ah, love, sweet love . . .

Well, not exactly.

More like food, glorious food. Chili dogs or caviar, McDonald's or Ma Maison, the anticipation, the craving, the savoring of food, can be as seductive and irresistible as a new love.

It's just that nine times out of ten, the relationship—with food—lasts longer.

Evidence of food seduction can be traced back as far as Adam and Eve, though personally I find it hard to swallow that two otherwise intelligent adults would commit sin over something as stupid as a red delicious. Now, had it been a cheeseburger, fries, and a shake . . .

Statistics show that the average person ingests about a ton of food each year. For many of us, a quarter of our income is spent to please our palates. Cookbooks fill the best-seller lists. Images of popular treats are reproduced on T-shirts, greeting cards, jigsaw puzzles, calendars, and tote bags. We greet each other with "Have you eaten?" more often than "Hello." We talk about food before we eat, while we are eating, and after we have eaten. It is a national obsession.

But pigging out is more than overeating. It is knowing how to pig, where to pig, who pigs, and what to do after pigging. Properly done, continually perfected, it is an art.

A warning: This book is not intended for those who eat "when I don't forget," or "if I have the time."* Rather, it is for those of us who, if given the choice between sex and a pound of chocolate chip cookies, would have to think twice before answering.

*The Surgeon General has determined this book might be hazardous to your health.

PART I

A HISTORY OF PIGGING OUT

I HAVE NOT YET BEGUN TO EAT...

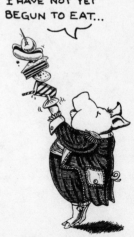

INTRODUCTION

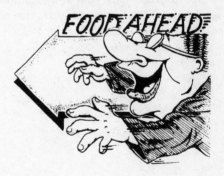

he time of day doesn't matter. You walk down any street, passing numerous store windows. Everywhere you turn, food awaits you in huge, wondrous quantities. Thirty-one flavors. Foot-long submarines. Double-layer devil's food cake.

You look twice but round the corner. The air smells like cake icing. Display cases groan with the weight of fresh baked goods. Giant neon burgers dance in circles above your head. A chocolate-chip cookie calls your name.

Suddenly, that uncontrollable desire overwhelms you. You move quickly. You wolf down a rare roast beef sandwich swimming au jus. You rejoice in a platter of French fries so greasy that your fingers become slick. You lose count by your seventh piece of pizza. You order one to go.

You are living proof that the only way to get rid of a temptation is to yield to it.

You are not alone.

Each year, America puts $2.5 billion into the economy in exchange for potato chips, pretzels, and popcorn alone.

Sara Lee sells forty-five thousand cheesecakes a day.

One out of every two meals is eaten out, and half of these—

whether breakfast, lunch, or dinner—are eaten in fast-food restaurants.

A billion Twinkies are devoured annually.

But pigging out is neither a recent trend nor an American phenomenon. Witness history. Pig-outs date back to the earliest recorded time: Roman orgies, Elizabethan banquets, Renaissance pleasure fairs. Even Marie Antoinette commanded, "Let them eat cake!" so she could lick the batter from the bowls.

Though a young country, America learned quickly. A lazy Indian woman, reluctant to go get water, instead boiled the venison she was preparing in some sap from a nearby maple; with this example in mind, trendy Pilgrims hastened pigging progress by smothering anything—fish, beef, poultry, beans (hence, Boston-baked beans)— in maple syrup. The overabundance of starch in the Colonists' diets so appalled the English governors that they repeatedly tried to introduce leafy green vegetables (which, in itself, seems reason enough for the later rebellion). And in the summer of 1790, George Washington, always the leader, ran up an ice-cream tab in excess of $200 (equivalent to at least $2,000 by today's economic standards) at a New York confectionery store.

All of which set the stage for . . .

GREAT MOMENTS IN PIG-OUT HISTORY

DATELINE: ***SARATOGA SPRINGS, NY, 1853.*** George Crum, the head chef at Moon's Lake House, is insulted when hotel-guest Cornelius Vanderbilt, the well-known railroad tycoon, sends back his dish of French fries, demanding that they be cut thinner and fried longer. In anger, Crum decides to teach the commodore a lesson and shaves off paper-thin slices of potatoes, throws them into a tub of ice water, lets them soak, and drops them in a vat of boiling grease. When they come out curled and fried crisp, he sprinkles salt on them and sends the potatoes back to the Vanderbilt table. Crum is bowled over when the guests send back their compliments and request another order. Soon, "Saratoga Chips" (later to become simply "potato chips") are a featured item on the hotel's menu.

DATELINE: ***PHILADELPHIA, PA, 1874.*** At the semicentennial celebration of the Franklin Institute, Robert Green sets up a concession selling a currently popular drink which consists of sweet cream, syrup, and carbonated soda. When he runs out of cream and begins to substitute vanilla ice cream, his "ice-cream soda" not only wins customer approval, but he sees his sales jump from $6 to $600 a day.

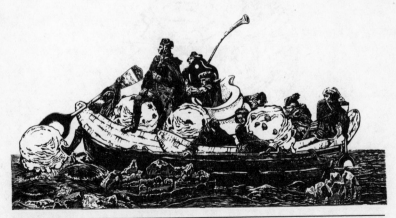

DATELINE: *ST. LOUIS, MO. 1890.* Concerned about the nutrition of his elderly, toothless patients, a Missouri physician uses peanuts to concoct a health-food product which is both high in protein and easily digestible. His "peanut butter" reaches even greater heights in Pennsylvania in 1923, when H. B. Reese, a former employee of the Hershey Company, combines it with chocolate and begins producing his soon-to-be-famous peanut butter cup.

DATELINE: *ST. LOUIS, MO. 1904.* At the World's Fair, Ernest Hamwi opens up a concession to sell zalabia, a crisp, waferlike Persian pastry baked on a flat waffle iron and topped with sugar, fruit, or other sweets. The stand next to Hamwi's offers ice cream in five- and ten-cent dishes. When one day business is extremely brisk and the ice-cream vendor runs out of glass cups, the quick-thinking Hamwi rolls one of his wafers into a cornucopia, lets it cool, and then scoops the ice cream into its mouth. The ice-cream cone is an immediate hit, and Hamwi happily struggles to keep up with the demand.

Also at the World's Fair, a Bavarian concessionaire, Anton Feuchtwanger, loans white gloves to his customers so that they can pick up the piping-hot sausages he is selling. But

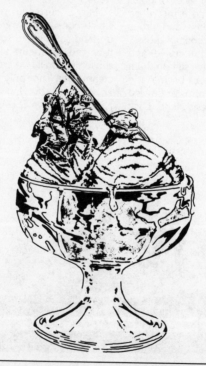

A HISTORY OF PIGGING OUT

when most of the patrons walk off with the gloves, his supply runs low, so Feuchtwanger talks his brother-in-law, a baker, into improvising a long, soft roll that can hold the meat . . . and thus, the first assemblage of the hot dog as we know it.

DATELINE: *NORTHERN CALIFORNIA, 1905.* Eleven-year-old Frank Epperson mixes up some popular soda-water powder and inadvertently leaves it outside overnight. When he awakes the next morning, he finds the stirring stick frozen upright in his drink and proudly shows his friends this unique "soda on a stick." Eighteen years later, in 1923, Epperson patents the Popsicle.

DATELINE: *PHILADELPHIA, PA, 1912.* The Whitman Candy Company, makers of the ever-popular Whitman's Sampler, introduces a new box with a chartlike guide printed on the inside of its lid, identifying which chocolate is which and finally putting an end to lousy guesses and punched-out centers.

DATELINE: *CHICAGO, IL, 1930.* On the heels of the stock-market crash and looking to become more cost-efficient, the Continental Baking Company grows concerned that the individual aluminum pans—used to make their "Little Short Cake Fingers" for the summer strawberry season—go unused for the remainder of the year. Determined to take advantage of the existing cake's popularity and make it profitable a full twelve months instead of three, Jimmy Dewar, a company manager, comes up with the idea of injecting the small sponge cake with a creamy filling.

Inspired by a billboard for "Twinkle Toe Shoes," he names his new cake "Twinkies."

DATELINE: *WHITMAN, MA, 1930.* Hotel owner Ruth Wakefield is experimenting with a favorite colonial cookie recipe when, lacking powdered cocoa, she decides to drop tiny bits of chopped chocolate into the batter. As the cookies bake, Mrs. Wakefield is surprised that the chocolate pieces do not melt as she had expecxted, but hold their shape, softening only slightly to a creamy texture. She serves the cookies anyway, naming them Toll House after the inn she owns. Her recipe catches on, and in 1939, the Nestlé Company (whose chocolate Mrs. Wakefield used) revolutionizes the cookie-baking market when it introduces semi-sweet "chocolate chips" in a convenient, ready-to-use package.

DATELINE: *CONNECTICUT, 1937.* Margaret Rudkin starts baking whole wheat bread with natural ingredients for a son who suffers from allergies. The bread is so delicious that doctors begin ordering it for themselves as well as their patients. A substantial mail-order business follows and Pepperidge Farm is on its way.

DATELINE: *NEWARK, NJ, 1941.* Forrest Mars, whose father Frank founded Mars Candies in 1920, starts his own chocolate company with an associate, Bruce Murrie. They combine their initials (M & M) to name their first product, a button-shaped, pill-sized candy created for the U.S. military because it could hold up in GI's pockets and rucksacks and be eaten without their trigger fingers getting sticky.

What's In a Name?

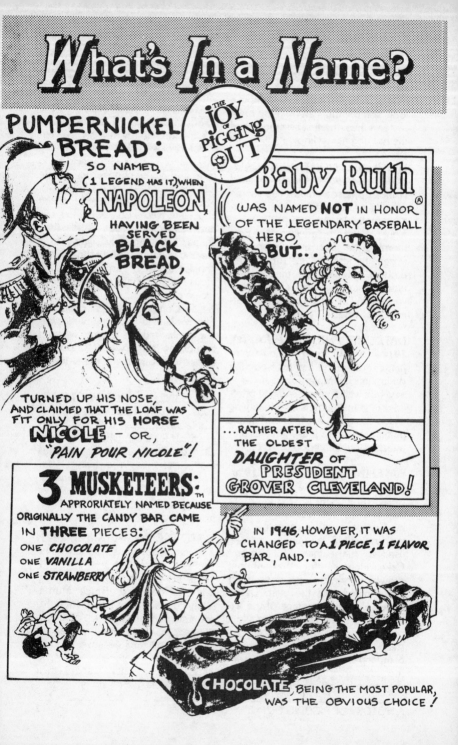

THE JOY OF PIGGING OUT

PUMPERNICKEL BREAD: SO NAMED, (1 LEGEND HAS IT), WHEN **NAPOLEON**, HAVING BEEN SERVED **BLACK BREAD**,

TURNED UP HIS NOSE, AND CLAIMED THAT THE LOAF WAS FIT ONLY FOR HIS **HORSE NICOLE** — OR, "PAIN POUR NICOLE"!

Baby Ruth® WAS NAMED **NOT** IN HONOR OF THE LEGENDARY BASEBALL HERO, **BUT...**

...RATHER AFTER THE OLDEST **DAUGHTER** OF **PRESIDENT GROVER CLEVELAND!**

3 MUSKETEERS:™ APPRORIATELY NAMED BECAUSE ORIGINALLY THE CANDY BAR CAME IN **THREE** PIECES: ONE *CHOCOLATE* ONE *VANILLA* ONE *STRAWBERRY*

IN 1946, HOWEVER, IT WAS CHANGED TO A **1 PIECE, 1 FLAVOR** BAR, AND...

CHOCOLATE, BEING THE MOST POPULAR, WAS THE OBVIOUS CHOICE!

HOT DOG. In 1901, on a chilly April day at the New York Polo Grounds, concessionaire Harry Stevens found himself losing money selling ice cream and cold sodas. He sent his salesmen out to find a product more desirable considering the weather conditions, and within an hour he had all his vendors hawking hot sausages (called "dachshunds") from portable hot-water tanks. In the press box, sports cartoonist Ted Dorgan was nearing his deadline, hard-pressed for an idea. Hearing Steven's vendors ("Hot dachshunds! Get your red-hot dachshunds!") he quickly drew a picture of sausages barking. But not sure how to spell "dachshund," he simply called them hot "dogs." The cartoon was a success and the name caught on.

HYDROX. No documentation exists, but it is believed that the name came about as a combination of the earth's two purest ingredients, hydrogen and oxygen. Others speculate that because the cookie's cream center was a dairy product and needed refrigeration, it was named after an English term for icebox. A third theory follows the thought that Hydrox is a contrived name—an acronym—derived from recipe code designations, with each letter representing a different ingredient.*

LORNA DOONE. In 1912, Nabisco was to introduce a British-type shortbread cookie called Hostess Jumbles. But it was when the name was later changed to Lorna Doone, after the heroine of Richard Blackmore's best-selling romance novel, that sales really took off.

TOOTSIE ROLL. Named by creator Leo Hirschfield for his daughter, Clara "Tootsie" Hirschfield.

ORANGE JULIUS. In 1926, real estate broker Bill Hamlin found the perfect spot in downtown Los Angeles for Julius Freed, a friend who wanted to open up an orange-juice stand. A would-be chemist, Hamlin was convinced he could add ingredients to fresh orange juice that would liven up the taste and thereby increase Freed's sales. Within four weeks, he concocted an "orange drink" made up of juice and purefood ingredients. Sales skyrocketed. Customers wanting the new drink would come to Freed's stand and ask, "How about an orange, Julius?" The name stuck.

---

*The early bird doesn't always catch the worm. While Hydrox is the Sunshine Biscuit Company's leading cookie, it is often looked upon as a carbon copy of the Nabisco Oreo, when in fact the Hydrox was marketed first—in 1908, some four years *before* the Oreo. What went wrong? Nobody knows for sure, but some industry spectators blame it on the name, and today the Oreo, the world's number-one-selling cookie, outsells the Hydrox approximately three to one.

HISTORIC PIGGING

"You Never Forget the First Time"

A look at some famous pig-out foods and places, and the year they started to make them.

1880 Thomas' English Muffins	1923 Milky Way
1886 Coca-Cola	1928 Peter Pan Peanut Butter
1888 Pastrami on rye (to go), (at Sussman Volk's Delancey St. Delicatessen)	1930 Snickers
	1932 Fritos
1896 Cracker Jack	1940 Dairy Queen (Joliet, IL)
1902 Animal Crackers	1940 Rice Krispies Marshmallow Treats
1907 Hershey's Kisses	1945 Baskin-Robbins (Glendale, CA)
1915 Velveeta	1948 Nestlé Quik
1919 A & W Rootbeer (Lodi, CA)	1948 McDonald's (original), 1948 (Pasadena, CA) (franchise), 1955 (Des Plaines, IL)
1921 Wise Potato Chips	
1921 Eskimo Pie	1949 Sara Lee Cheesecake
1921 Mounds	1950 Kellogg's Sugar Pops†

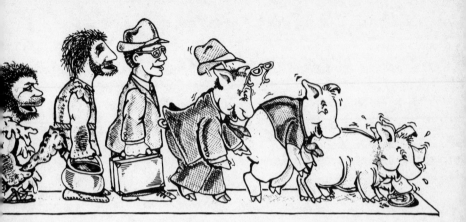

1953 Jell-O Instant Pudding

1954 Burger King (Miami, FL)

1958 Pizza Hut (Wichita, KA)

1958 International House of Pancakes (North Hollywood, CA)

1968 Big Mac*

1975 Famous Amos Chocolate Chip Cookie (Los Angeles, CA)

1976 Häagen-Dazs Dip store (Brooklyn, NY)

1978 Reese's Pieces

1979 David's Cookies (New York, NY)

*Original cost: 49¢.
†First ready-sweetened, ready-to-eat breakfast cereal.

PART II

HOW TO PIG OUT

I'LL EAT TO THAT

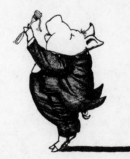

THE SIX BASIC FOOD GROUPS

he key to pigging out is a varied diet that includes portions of every kind of food desired. Researchers have translated piggers' needs and preferences into an easy-to-use guide for food selection, sorting food into six groups on the basis of its availability, content, and method of preparation. (No group claims to make a noteworthy contribution to any diet whatsoever.) Following are the six basic groups and the chief foods found in each. Recommended daily servings vary, but as a rule of thumb, remember: Nothing succeeds like excess.

THE SIX BASIC FOOD GROUPS*

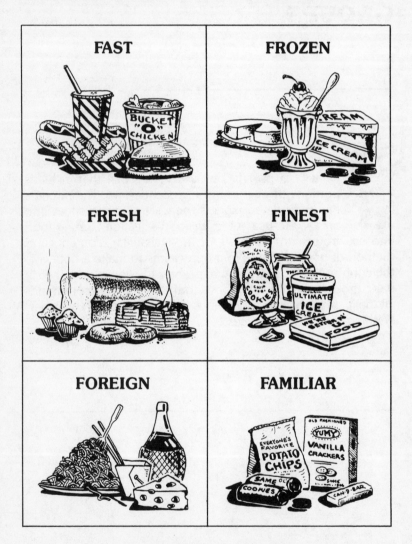

FAST

FROZEN

FRESH

FINEST

FOREIGN

FAMILIAR

*Fruits, vegetables, and vitamins are not discussed because unless dipped in chocolate their relationship to pigging out has yet to be determined.

Group 1. FAST. This group provides the main staples of the pigger's diet: hamburgers, cheeseburgers (double cheeseburgers, chili cheeseburgers, bacon cheeseburgers), fries, onion rings, submarines (hoagies, heroes, poorboys, cheesesteaks), hot dogs (chili dogs, cheese dogs, footlongs), fried chicken, fish 'n' chips, barbecued ribs.

Group 2. FROZEN. The major components of this group are milk by-products: ice cream, sundaes, shakes, malts, floats, splits, bonbons, and Fudgsicles. Also includes raw Pillsbury chocolate-chip cookie dough, Mystic Mints (only after left in the freezer a minimum of two hours), Milky Ways (ditto), Stouffer's Lasagna, Mrs. Paul's Fish Sticks, Rich's Bavarian Creme Puffs, Ore-Ida Tater Tots, and all Sara Lee cheesecakes.

Group 3: FRESH. As in freshly *baked:* pizza, cookies, cakes, brownies, pies, bagels, doughnuts, bear claws, sticky buns, cinnamon rolls, pancakes, napoleons, éclairs, and all French, rye, sourdough, and Italian breads.

Group 4. FINEST. Designer foods for the pretentious pigger: Häagen-Dazs, Famous Amos, David's, Godiva, Krön, Orville Redenbacher's, Jelly Bellys, Gourmet Mints, as well as old standards—lox, Brie, caviar,* prosciutto.

Group 5: FOREIGN. This group provides the pigger with the continental eating experience: croissants, crumpets, tacos, tamales, tostadas, spaghetti, ravioli, linguine, vermicelli, cannoli, knishes, chopped liver, sushi, fried dumplings, and anything else Chinese. As alternatives, foreign foods such as English muffins, French toast, Turkish taffy, Belgian waffles, and German chocolate cake may be substituted.

Group 6. FAMILIAR. The fun foods (which the pigger has most often been denied or forced to eat in secret): M & M's, Snickers, Hershey bars, Suzy Q's, Ding Dongs, Twinkies, Devil Dogs, Yodels, Zingers, Tastykakes, Oreos, Mallomars, Raisinets, Milanos, Fritos, Chee-Tos, Cracker Jack, Velveeta, Pringles, Pop Tarts, Vienna Fingers, Corn Nuts, Beer Nuts, caramel corn, and cinnamon-covered graham crackers, to name a few.

---

*Caviar was not thought to be much of a luxury in the seventeenth century. Consider an old Italian proverb, "Chi mangia di caviale/mangia moschi, merdi, e sale," which translates, "He who eats caviar/eats flies, shit, and salt."

RULES FOR PIGGING ETIQUETTE

Proper pigging includes not only a diet of foods from each of the six groups, but requires an understanding of basic etiquette. Before we can examine where to pig, there are a few rules one should know concerning how to pig.

RULE: If God had meant man to use a knife and a fork, he wouldn't have given him fingers.

As a pigging utensil, the combination of the fore- and middle fingers is unbeatable. Use it. Scoop with it, taste with it, pick with it. Do not allow previous table training to interfere with your enjoyment. Remember, most pigging out is done alone, or in secret, so no one else is there to see what you are doing. If others are present, chances are they will be too busy eating to notice; and, even if they do, you will be having too much fun to care.

NO

YES

RULE: If you don't pick, wolf.

Picking is more fun: picking the icing off a cake, picking the raisins from a box of Raisin Bran, picking out the red gummy bears. Picking gets you exactly what you want or lets you have a taste of everything. It also helps you convince yourself you're not really eating.

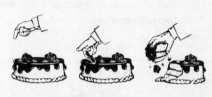

PICKING　　　**WOLFING**

Wolfing, on the other hand, is more gratifying. There's no turning back. You've wanted something for so long that you can't stand it anymore and you have to have as much of it in your mouth as possible. Wolfing does not work well with the more delicate foods, such as chocolates or hors d'oeuvres. With the right cheeseburger, however, it is heaven.

RULE: Try to pig in a standing position.

Although this is virtually impossible in a sit-down restaurant (unless you have very short legs), pigging out over a sink or in front of an opened refrigerator is guaranteed to enhance your eating pleasure. Additionally, calories don't count until you are seated at the table, in front of the TV, or in bed.

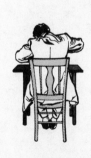
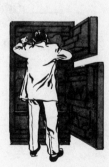

WRONG　　　**RIGHT**

RULE: No food is bad cold.

Pasta, pizza, cookies, candy bars, brownies—foods normally eaten hot or at room temperature are even better after spending the night in the refrigerator.

GOOD

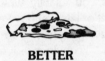

BETTER

RULE: Never trust a blue food.

No matter how hungry, it just might be your last.

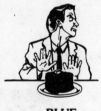

BLUE

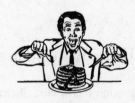

NOT BLUE

HOW TO EAT A . . .

Jelly Doughnut: Scoop out jelly with spoon. Eat. Stuff inside with miniature Reese's Peanut Butter Cups. Warm in oven.

Mallomar: Pick off chocolate coating. Suck out marshmallow middle. Pop graham wafer in mouth.

Cheesecake: Say, "I'll only have a sliver." Eat. Cut another sliver. Eat. Continue until cake is gone. Smile demurely.

Smorgasbord: Grab the largest plate. Bypass the jellied aspic molds and head straight for the desserts (these go quickly). Keep hot and cold foods separate. Avoid diners with blue hair or those dressed in polyester. They dawdle, have difficulty deciding, and move slowly.

Chocolate Pudding: Cut pudding with spoon, puncturing skin. Tunnel pudding out of dish, leaving skin in place. When pudding has been eaten, wrap skin around spoon. Hold spoon vertically and scrape skin off with teeth.

Pizza: Cut into pie-shaped wedge (large). Crack slice in middle and eat with the sides curled up to avoid losing the filling. Do not even think of using a knife and fork.

Barbecued Ribs: Let grease drip to elbow. Do not wipe mouth between bites.

Milano: Insert one-half of cookie in mouth. Apply pressure with both upper and bottom teeth to center of cookie. Without biting through, slowly pull cookie out of mouth, scraping off brown-edged wafer but leaving chocolate middle intact. Repeat with other half. Let remaining chocolate melt in mouth. (See also diagram p. 22: How to Open a Bag of Pepperidge Farm Cookies.)

The last cookie, the last cracker, the last piece of candy: Look both ways. In one continuous motion, scoop up cookie (or cracker, or candy) and stuff in mouth before someone else can beat you to it.

How to OPEN A BAG OF PEPPERIDGE FARM COOKIES

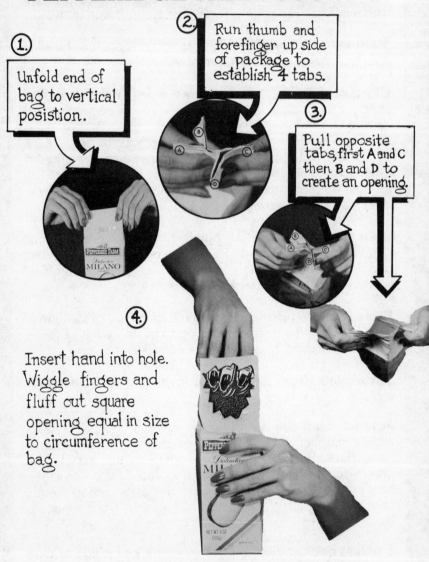

1. Unfold end of bag to vertical posistion.

2. Run thumb and forefinger up side of package to establish 4 tabs.

3. Pull opposite tabs, first A and C then B and D to create an opening.

4. Insert hand into hole. Wiggle fingers and fluff out square opening equal in size to circumference of bag.

Pepperidge Farm cookies come packaged in bags with three (3) layers, each layer containing a paper cup with a minimum of five (5) cookies (as in the Milano) and a maximum of nine (9) cookies (the Orleans). Proper pigging dictates that at least one full cup must be consumed in one sitting.

'TIS THE SEASON TO PIG OUT:

A Guide to Holiday Pigging

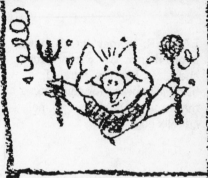

THANKSGIVING: The most famous pig-out in history. The fact that it marked the introduction of popcorn is reason enough for celebration. But you really are thankful. Thankful for the turkey, thankful for the pumpkin pie, thankful for the marshmallows on top of the sweet potatoes, and thankful for the leftovers that taste even better cold.

CHRISTMAS: The holiday that finds you surrounded by those you love most: ham, turkey, roast beef, sugar cookies, gingerbread, plum pudding, candy canes, and eggnog. If giving a gift in person, it is always best to give something edible; on opening, the recipient will feel obligated to share the contents with you.

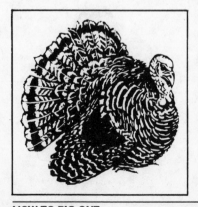

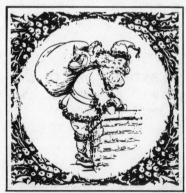

EASTER: Forget the Sunday family dinner. We're talking milk chocolate bunnies here. Trade black jelly beans for little sister's marshmallow chickens and malted milk eggs.

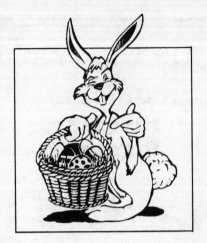

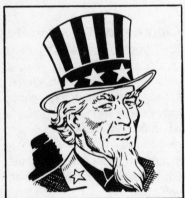

FOURTH OF JULY (also MEMORIAL DAY, LABOR DAY): The all-American pig-out—hamburgers, hot dogs, and apple pie. For guilt-ridden piggers needing an excuse, this is it. You're doing it for your country.

VALENTINE'S DAY: Of course you'll be their valentine. You'll do anything for chocolate.

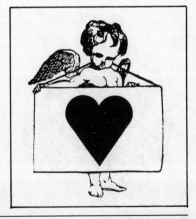

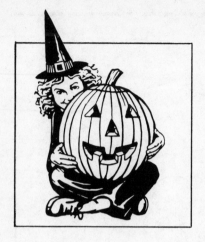

HALLOWEEN: The pigger's dream come true: free candy.

JEWISH HOLIDAYS: Dates vary, but do your best to wangle an invitation to either a Passover or Rosh Hashanah dinner. Where there are Jews, there's good food. Plenty of it.

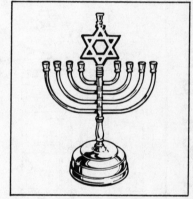

THE PIG-OUT KITCHEN
What's Cookin', Good-Lookin'?

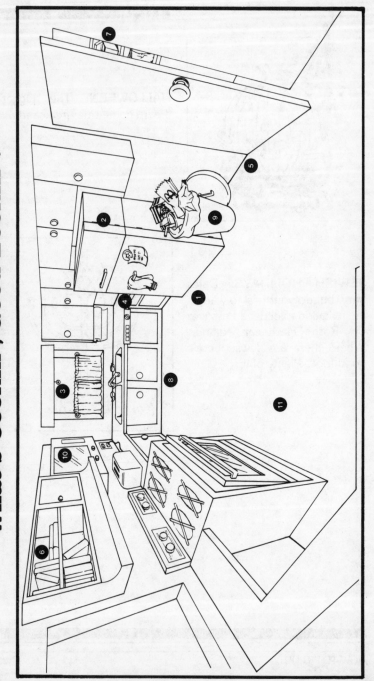

The kitchen is, of course, the pigger's sanctuary. Yet it is important to note that the typical pig-out kitchen is not necessarily identified by well-stocked pantry shelves, a refrigerator filled to the brim, a stove in constant use, or a compilation of the latest gadgets. While any of these characteristics is certainly advantageous and should not be dismissed, the following list of eleven identifying signals is the real guide.

1. Faded from overexposure to light—a result of repeated opening and closing of refrigerator door.

2. Loose hinges (see #1 above).

3. Black-out shades so neighbors can't see what you are doing.

4. Silverware tray. Contains hacksaw (for cutting frozen brownies), a complete set of bent spoons (from eating ice cream directly out of the carton), and rubber spatula (to get every last drop).

5. Absence of dog, cat, or any other pet that could lick up crumbs faster than you.

6. Complete set of local telephone directories (as well as menus from neighborhood restaurants) for ordering out.

7. Regional Goodie Shelf. Enables immediate identification of geographical location by particular brands housed—Entenmann's, Drake's Cakes, Tastykakes, Wise Potato Chips (East); Freihoeffer's cookies (upstate New York); Jay's Potato Chips (Midwest); See's Candies, Van de Kamp's (West); Krispy Kreme doughnuts (South); Sanders Hot Fudge (Detroit).

8. Permanent indentations (à la Grauman's Chinese Theatre) caused by regular pigging while hovering over sink.

9. How is it that what can fill a ten-gallon capacity trash can cannot fulfill a one-quart-capacity stomach?

10. For warming up boxes of White Castle hamburgers ordered through the mail (see HOW TO PIG OUT: Mail-Order Pig-Out).

11. A floor so clean you can eat off it—and often do.

HOW TO PIG OUT WHEN THERE'S NOTHING IN THE HOUSE

It is unconstitutional to walk to the refrigerator, open both doors, stare at $250 worth of groceries, and declare, "There's nothing to eat." It is an even greater sacrilege to open the doors, find nothing but condiments and staples, and voice the same sentiment. Most kitchens, even when in the nothing-in-the-house state, include three deceptively simple "basics" which provide the pigger with a multitude of gastronomic pleasures.

WHITE BREAD

If there is one food that is the desperate pigger's saving grace, it is bread. True bread, of course. White bread. From its moist, foam-rubber texture to its secret dough conditioners.

One of the nicest things about bread is that it can be eaten many ways: plain, toasted, or topped. If you are eating bread plain, besides smearing it with butter, peanut butter, or preserves, you may prefer this childhood delight: cut off the crusts, roll the rest into a ball, and pop it straight into your mouth. (Or try dipping the ball into some melted butter first, then rolling it in Parmesan cheese and toasting the whole thing in the broiler.) For those who savor the crust, the reverse is recommended. Using the rim of a Dixie cup, punch a hole in the center of the bread; after eating—er, removing—the hole, toss the slice into a frying pan, add a pat of butter, and cook an egg in the middle.

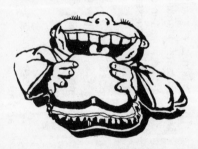

Toasted, bread can be seasoned with herbs, then toasted again, to make a giant crouton. Or before toasting, sprinkle the bread with some instant hot cocoa mix and—presto!—pain au chocolat. Lastly, toast can be topped with a mixture of cream cheese, vanilla, cinnamon, and sugar to make a treat that almost tastes like cheesecake.

PEANUT BUTTER

More than any other food, piggers take an adamant stand on peanut butter. They either love it or they hate it. There's no middle ground, except for the group of die-hard purists who resent the substance simply for its high nutritional value.

Peanut butter is a pleasure if solely for the many ways one can eat it. The most common method is to spread it on bread, toast, and crackers (with or without jelly), on apples and bananas, and even—as a last resort—on celery. A second technique—an obvious one, but for some reason less-known—is to eat it with a spoon. If you are using a spoon, it is suggested that you dip twice; first into the peanut butter and then into one of many "toppings" such as jam, jelly, honey, instant cocoa mix, or sugar. With a spoon, peanut butter can also be eaten

from a bowl, where it is at its best mixed with a little milk and powdered sugar, producing a substance not entirely unlike cake icing.

Still, as dedicated piggers know, the best way to eat peanut butter is the simplest: using the finger—a longtime favorite and heartily recommended for the oral sensuality it provides (see HOW TO PIG OUT: Rules for Pigging Etiquette, Rule #1).

THE TELEPHONE

Ultimately, if "nothing in the house" really means that there is *nothing* in the house, the pigger can turn to the telephone. A number of local stores and restaurants offer quick delivery of pizza, chicken, Chinese food, and groceries.* And should nothing in the house also mean that there's no money in the house (and Pizza Man doesn't take credit cards and the Chicken Shack—which does—is closed), don't despair. When all else fails, send yourself a Candygram.

---

*Lucky New Yorkers. The Burger Joint (two Manhattan locations) offers a pigger's dream: an emergency "Burger Hotline," with free delivery of eight-ounce char-broiled burgers until 3:00 A.M.

MAIL-ORDER PIG-OUT

Because many of the best pig-out foods are regional specialties or products of Mom-and-Pop operations, your supermarket isn't able to carry them all. Luckily, your mailman is. While a number of catalogues offer live Maine lobsters, Texas-sized steaks, and Wisconsin cheeses, the following list contains some one-of-a-kind exceptional edibles that can be purchased through the mail. So relax, Peoria, real New York cheesecake is only a postcard away.

CHEESECAKE. *Junior's,* 386 Flatbush Avenue, Brooklyn, NY (212) 852-5257. (See also WHERE TO PIG OUT: A "Deli" Guide to New York.) The cream of New York cheesecakes from a town that knows of cheesecake. Large size only; serves ten to twelve slices (one person).

WHITE CASTLE HAMBURG-ERS. For the uninitiated, these East Coast and Midwest white-tiled hamburger stands are, to many, heaven on earth. They're always open and at just over two bits a burger, always a deal. They have no clowns, no catchy jingles, no signs touting how many billion sold. What they do have—what piggers flock here for—are cheap, greasy burgers, square in shape and with holes in them.

The big news is that White Castle hamburgers are now available for shipping. Because they are steamed, not fried, they are perfect for a microwave (microwaves work best with products prepared at high moisture levels). At the regular store price (plus handling costs), hundreds of these pig-out morsels can be packed in dry ice and in your hands within thirty-six hours. The only things you'll be missing are those wonderful company newsletters announcing who's back from vacation, who's having a birthday, and who's been voted "Bun Burner of the Week." Call 1-(800)-W-CAS-TLE.

KENTUCKY BOURBON BALLS. *Rebecca-Ruth Candies,* P.O. Box 64, Frankfort, KY 40602 (or visit the retail stores in Lexington, Louisville, and Woodford County). This old-fashioned candy company was started by two former schoolteachers, and the delicious chocolates are the kind your grandmother would make—if Granny kept a bottle of 100-proof Kentucky bourbon next to the mixing bowl. This Kentucky colonel isn't a fried-chicken magnate but a soft bourbon cream dipped in thin, dark chocolate and topped with a pecan. Unfortunately, for anyone living outside Kentucky these unusual candies can't be mailed, since the federal authorities don't permit more than .5 percent alcohol in candy and Rebecca-Ruth bourbon balls contain close to 2 percent. But short of hopping the next plane to bluegrass country, what you can do (no, what you *should* do) is send for the rum- and crème de menthe-flavored chocolates— which the gang at the post office will let by. You see, these two liquors have a stronger taste than bourbon, so it doesn't take as much to flavor the candy. . . .

SALTWATER TAFFY. *Forbes Candies,* P.O. Box 270, Virginia Beach, VA 23458. Why wait for summer or until you can afford a house on the beach to enjoy these boardwalk goodies? Available in both one- and two-pound boxes of assorted flavors, they're the next best thing to being there.

BEEF SALAMI. *Katz's Delicatessen,* 205 E. Houston Street, New York, NY (see WHERE TO PIG OUT: A "Deli" Guide to New York). As the sign in this Lower East Side landmark says, "Send a salami to your boy in the army." Or, better yet, send it to yourself.

CHOCOLATE-COVERED CARA-MELS. *Fun in the Sun Candies,* 232 North Palm Canyon Drive, Palm Springs, CA 92262. Maybe it's the giant, Oldenburg-like candy cane that sits outside the white stucco shop. Or maybe it's the enthusiastic, mouth-watering way the owner describes the stacks of boxes of homemade candies. Or maybe it's just because this store is neither selling a well-known brand nor is part of a chain. Whatever the case, the chocolate-covered caramels—in seven different flavors—are a pigger's delight. (Open from November

to March 15 only; the rest of the year, "the li'l ole candy maker" closes shop to research and perfect new delicacies that he can add to his stock in the future.)

BEIGNETS. *Cafe du Monde,* 813 Decatur Street, New Orleans, LA 70116 (see WHERE TO PIG OUT: The Hole Truth). These French Quarter, French Market, French doughnuts don't exactly come ready to eat, but everything you need to make about six dozen of the delicious square pastries is packed inside this two-pound box. Pass the powdered sugar.

SMITHFIELD HAM. *Gwaltney of Smithfield,* 115 Brand Road, Salem, VA 24156 (703) 387-2120. This lean, cured country ham (available from eight to fifteen pounds) is a Virginia classic that'll make your taste buds stand up and take notice.

GOO GOO CLUSTERS. *Standard Candy Company,* P.O. Box 101025, Nashville, TN 37210. "A good ole Southern treat." If you haven't heard of Goo Goos, you probably haven't been listening to the Grand Ole Opry and you definitely haven't been to Tennessee. But don't despair; let Tennessee come to you—in boxes of six, twelve, or twenty-four. Exactly what is a Goo Goo Cluster? Said to be "the South's favorite candy," it's a round mound of chocolate, peanuts, caramel, and marshmallow. And definitely addicting. (Gourmet piggers may wish to try the new Goo Goo Supreme, made with pecans instead of peanuts.)

PART III

WHERE TO PIG OUT

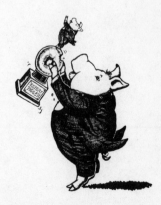

AUTHOR'S NOTE:

The viewpoints in this section are entirely subjective and only meant to reflect an expert's opinion.

HOW TO SPOT A
GOOD PIG-OUT PLACE

n the road again? Well, say good-bye to those endless hours of thumbing through phone books and riding around with your stomach growling. For piggers away from home—be it three miles or three thousand—here is a quick and easy lesson in how to seek out the best of pig-out restaurants.

THE LOOK.—Give the place a second glance if the neon sign (its lights having blown out ages ago) says "Coffee Shop," "Diner," "Luncheonette," "Grill," or, more to the point, just "EAT." Stop immediately, then run—fast—if the building has character, the lighting has the right glare, and the counter is chrome and Formica. The joint can fit any of a battery of names—dive, shack, out-of-the-way, hole-in-the-wall—but only one adjective: classic. While the best of the lot sport a somewhat time-worn look, remember new isn't necessarily bad, nor necessarily more expensive. Better to be wary of the unassuming pig-out place that develops a following, expands, and remodels, only to become as undistinguished as the ferns that line the walls; or of an overemphasis on gimmick and decor. Unless, of course, you can *eat* the decor. . . .

Give extra points for customers waiting patiently in line. Chances are if they're not complaining they're regulars who know that what they're getting is worth the wait. An old-fashioned Hamilton Beach milk-shake mixer is also a good sign.

THE SERVICE.—Real waitresses have names like Betty and Dixie. They wear matching uniforms, but never costumes. They're slightly older. They bristle and bustle. They mother you a little and tease you a lot.

Though somewhat less common, waiters should have names like Joe and Phil and preferably be white-shirted, bow-tied, and middle-aged, with a butcher's apron to the floor. Check to see if they're at home behind the counter. If slinging plates, refilling coffee, dishing out dessert, and making change becomes a perfectly choreographed routine, damn the crowds and push your way through to the next available stool.

THE FOOD.—The right smell has to greet you when you walk through the door. Look to see that at least one of your favorite things is being served. (Anything "like mother used to make" probably isn't.) It's best to avoid multiple-choice, billboard-sized menus: too many specialties and nothing is special. A limited number of offerings is the safer bet. Only when each item is really outstanding will most places dare to do this. Threaten to kill if they don't save you the last piece of homemade pie or chocolate cake.

BEST BETS

THE HOLE TRUTH

Powdered, glazed, chocolate-covered, cream-filled, coconut-flaked. The doughnut is, in its infinite variety, the ultimate pig-out food. Fried and made with globs of wonderful sugar, it is a double dose of decadence. And not unlike the ideal lover—rich, sensual, irresistibly desirable, and available twenty-four hours a day.

Down to basics. Pick off the topping, suck out the filling, and what you have left comes in two standard forms—soft and gummy, or well fried and crunchy. Staunch piggers will express clear preferences for one type over the other, and rarely will any group agree. Likewise, exactly how the doughnut got its hole is a subject for debate, although the consensus is that it had something to do with a man named Hansen Gregory.

Legend has it that Gregory, a Maine sea captain, was munching on fried cakes when a sudden storm blew through, forcing his ship off course. In an attempt to regain control, he grabbed for the wheel, inadvertently pushing the cake he was holding into one of the spokes, thereby creating a hole. Others claim that Gregory deliberately punched out the centers in order to make the cakes lighter (*after* he had lost six men overboard, the heaviness of the doughnuts having made them sink to the bottom and drown). Or maybe, some feel, it wasn't all that splashy: Gregory was merely busy at the helm when the ship's steward arrived with a plate of just-fried cakes. Too hot to hold, he quickly slipped them over the spokes to cool off and—voilà—a hole. (Still, there are piggers who feel that the hole had nothing to do with

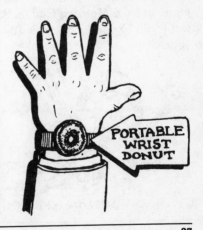

PORTABLE WRIST DONUT

Gregory. Rather, they purport, a Colonial woman was frying cakes in her kitchen when a drunken Indian came by, aimed an arrow through the window, and shot a hole in one of them.)

Whatever their origin, doughnuts have come a long way in the last 150 years. But with the ease of mixes, frozen dough, and thaw-and-serve brands, the chains and their franchise shops are trying to cover up with size (foot-long maple twists, eight-ounce apple fritters) what they sometimes lack in quality. All of which means a good doughnut is hard to find.

Make that *was*. **Stan's Corner Donut Shoppe** (10948 Weyburn Avenue, Los Angeles) offers gastronomic ecstasy in close to 100 variations, most notably their peanut-butter pocket, a raised dough-nut stuffed with peanut butter, heavily coated with chocolate icing, topped with chocolate chips, and so perfect it doesn't break, it tears. The doughnut selection at **Reeves Restaurant and Bakery** (see WHERE TO PIG OUT: The Top Ten) can be counted on one hand, but their blueberry—crumbly and cakey, with the fruit mixed right into the dough—is, in and of itself, reason to move to D.C. At **Mary Elizabeth's Cruller Bar** (6 East 37 Street, NYC) the sugar-and-cin-namon-dusted cake doughnuts, with their crisply fried edges, make dunking a new experience. Try to get there early, before the home-made honey buns sell out. But the king of doughnuts is undoubtedly **Cafe Du Monde**'s square-shaped French beignet—crunchy, chewy, light and tender, and buried in powdered sugar. Sold in groups of three, all night long, this is what a trip to New Orleans is all about (813 Decatur Street, in the French Market). And as long as you're in town, do as the locals do and head to the Lakeside Shopping Cen-ter, where the **Morning Call** (3325 Severn Avenue) fries up a per-fect (even bigger) beignet that (be still, my heart) you'll get to sugar yourself.

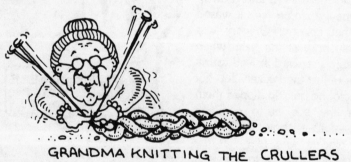

GRANDMA KNITTING THE CRULLERS

TOP DOG(S)

Manhattan hot-dog vendors offer customers stewed onions with their franks, but in Coney Island, it's sauerkraut that's optional. In Los Angeles, chili dogs are popular, loaded with mustard, onions, and sometimes grated cheese. Down South they serve up corn dogs—wieners dipped in batter and fried—while throughout the Midwest hot dogs are preferred slit down the middle, then wrapped in bacon and covered with melted cheese.

Clearly, hot dogs could be considered the pigger's geographical guide to the country, so *The Joy of Pigging Out* presents a guide to the country's best:

The genuine New York hot dog is still in its casing, tied at the end, and snaps when you bite it. **Nathan's** (Surf and Stillwell avenues, Brooklyn) sets the standard by which all others have been judged and is that rare pig-out place where the food lives up to the reputation. In Manhattan alone, there are over 3,000 licensed hot-dog vendors (most identified by the blue-and-orange umbrellas of **Sabrett**) but the best of the breed has got to be at **Katz's Delicatessen** (205 E. Houston Street), where the dogs are so extraordinary (both with and without sauerkraut) that when you bite them, they bite back. . . . In Los Angeles, it's dog-eat-dog, where **Pink's** (711 N. La Brea Avenue) and **Tail o' the Pup*** (311 N. La Cienega Blvd.) dish out the epitome of pig-out franks, so heavily—make that *heavenly*—laden with chili that you'll wonder where the dog went. But it's there. And even on its own, it tastes great. These long-standing favorites, however, are being challenged by a relative newcomer, **Pop Cuisine** (at **Heaven,** 10250 Santa Monica Blvd.), a fifties-style Woolworth's lunch counter tucked away in the back of a trendy gift and clothing store. The quarter-pounders here are plump and juicy, the hands-down winner in the flavor department, and come on a tasty whole wheat sesame seed bun. . . . Hot dog joints abound in Chicago, with their "Vienna" signs out front; while all may look similar, discriminating piggers know they're not. The blue ribbon goes to

---

*See also WHERE TO PIG OUT: What You See Is What You Get.

Poochie's (3832 Dempster, Skokie) where the "red hot"—boiled or steamed, but never grilled—is covered with condiments (mustard, chopped onions, sweet relish, sport peppers, sliced tomatoes, and a dill pickle spear) and nestled in what makes a Chicago hot dog special, one of Rosen's poppy-seed buns (steamed but never toasted). . . . If in Philadelphia, follow tradition and head to **Levis** (507 S. Sixth Street), an eighty-year-old luncheonette done in do-it-yourself paneling and neon yellow paint, where the hot dog is a hot dog, and one bite brings back a thousand memories. As does the terrific soda fountain offering the best in malts, shakes, floats, and cherry Cokes. . . . Though a hot-dog stand in a chic resort town like Palm Springs might seem to be a paradox, **McSorley's** (67795 Highway 111) manages to serve up one which is uniquely delicious, thanks to spicy mustard, a good dog, and an unbeatable "oven fresh roll," made of French bread that's warm and crusty but won't tear into the roof of your mouth when you bite it. Don't leave without checking out the homemade pies, cookies, and cinnamon rolls. Definitely worth a second look. . . . A note to piggers in all points in between: **Howard Johnson's** (everywhere) offers a hot dog that you'll swear didn't come from a chain. Their famous "finger roll"—a thick slice of white bread, grilled and buttered and fashioned to fit—is a pigging classic. And you thought they just made ice cream.

SELF-SERVE

A good cafeteria is hog heaven, appealing directly to the pigger's sense of greed. While the offerings may not be any more varied than those on a typical family-restaurant menu, the joy comes in having all that food out where you can see it—on the line—waiting just for you.

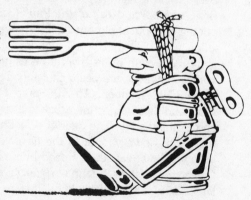

The Highland Park Cafeteria (4611 Cole, Dallas) is as American as the apple pie they serve. Pictures of the U.S. presidents, from Washington through Reagan, line the walls; details of "what's to eat" flash at you from overhead TV monitors instead of menu boards. (Working here definitely has its benefits; every recipe is tested by the staff before the public tastes it.) There is an incredibly varied selection of food, starting with seventeen salads, continuing through numerous entrees (many, like chicken and dumplings, or chicken-fried steak, are regional), and into the sweet stuff. Great homemade rolls, too. Besides the normal serving line, the Shakespeare Buffet is offered, where for a fixed price the cafeteria is turned into an all-you-can-eat smorgasbord. . . . *Miss Hulling's* (1103 Locust, St. Louis), with its cheerful pink-and-white decor and fresh flowers on the tables, looks more like a tearoom than the cafeteria it is. Standing out is a large selection of hot entrees, plus a daily special. The roast beef is always rare, carved for you on the spot; vegetables are fresh, not frozen. Don't miss the desserts, including the famous chocolate split, lemon split, and angel-food cakes. If you're too stuffed, they're also sold at the bakery next door, along with cookies, doughnuts, bread, and old-fashioned box lunches. . . . Cafeterias were once a Manhattan lunch and dinner staple, but now they're practically extinct. Which makes *Dubrow's* (515 Seventh Avenue) like a trip back to Old New York. It's well stocked with the basics—good soups, hearty entrees—and is packed with cabbies and workers from the nearby garment district. Desserts are oversized and tasty (although the whipped cream is straight from a can). . . . *Sholl's Cafeteria* (1433 K Street, N.W., Washington, D.C.) serves well-made, substantial food in a classic cafeteria setting. In a city certainly known for pinching *your* pennies, Sholl's fights to help piggers fight back. At no time is this more apparent than first thing in the morning, when breakfast is any combination of eggs, bacon, sausage, pancakes, and toast. What's so great is that you pay individually for each item (an egg, any style, is 20¢) and you can order any amount of any one you wish. . . . At *Clifton's* (numerous Los Angeles locations, including Century Square Shopping Center, Century City) it's always Thanksgiving, with a turkey dinner (white meat or dark, hand-carved, straight from the bird), including dressing, gravy, and cranberry sauce, available all day long, seven days a week. . . . Bright, stylish, and always busy, *The Commissary* (1710 Samson, Philadelphia) offers gourmet-style food at decent (but above-average-for-a-cafeteria) prices. The menu selections vary daily but include cold salads, smoked fish, charcuterie, omelets, pasta—and the world's best carrot cake.

THE BIG TEN

Football? You've got to be kidding. These schools score big where it *really* counts.

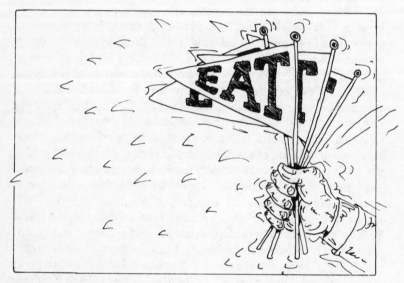

1.–GEORGIA TECH:—
The Varsity (61 North Avenue, N.W., Atlanta). This huge drive-in (it has a multilevel parking lot) serves fifteen thousand piggers a day and sells more Coca-Cola than any other single retail outlet in the world. Hamburgers and hot dogs are assembled to order, in mass-production style, on a conveyor belt behind a long, stainless-steel counter. The fries and onion rings are exquisitely greasy delights. Enjoy them in any of the five "dining" rooms, each containing a TV set tuned to a different channel. Imagine. Pigging out and *All My Children*, too.

2.–UNIVERSITY OF MICHIGAN:—*Drake's* (709 N. University, Ann Arbor). A dimly lit combination sandwich shop, soda fountain, tearoom, candy store, and campus institution, where little has changed since it first opened in 1929. The ritual is simple: You write your own order (using what has to be the world's tiniest pencil), fetch it when it's ready, and linger as

long as you like. The milk shakes pay homage to days gone by, courtesy of real ice cream and homemade chocolate syrup. The perfect escape from the worry of last-minute cramming and overdue papers.

3.–CORNELL UNIVERSITY: —*Noyes Lodge* (on campus, Ithaca, NY). *On campus?* It might sound odd, but anyone who has either gone to or visited Cornell knows that (thanks to the School of Hotel and Restaurant Management) Cornell has, quite simply, the best campus food in the country. It's the college pigger's dream: Each dining unit has its own kitchen (there's no central commissary here), so there's no chance you'll be getting a mass-produced meal or last week's leftovers. Noyes Lodge, overlooking Beebe Lake and Triphammer Falls, features waiter service and an award-winning menu of burgers, salads, omelets, quiche, and sandwiches. The university also has its own bakery (they deliver), its own ice cream, even its own milk. Get your transcript and application ready.

4–UNIVERSITY OF TEXAS:—*The Hoffbrau* (613 W. Sixth Street, Austin). A steak-and-potatoes hole in the wall whose incredible popularity has spawned a host of (good) imitators near campuses throughout the state. Still, there's none quite like the original.

5.–INDIANA UNIVERSITY:— *Mother Bear's* (428 E. Third, Bloomington). This is a town with a pizza place on practically every corner, but Mother Bear's stands head and shoulders above the rest, attracting huge lines every night and dishing out a pie well worth the extra weight. The sauce—fiery and hot due to crushed red and black peppers—is the very stuff a great pig-out is made of.

6.–UNIVERSITY OF COLORADO:—*Dot's Diner* (799 Pearl, Boulder). College students may not be known for their discriminating palates, but locals line up here, too. A classic dive, housed in a Sinclair gas station and serving the best of diner food: breakfast and lunch, with the emphasis on the eggs. There's a different omelet every day (depending on what fresh veggies are in stock), good *huevos,* and an oven-baked German pancake. The grits and gravy are a refreshing change from the typical Colorado menu of sprouts and smoothies.

7.–HARVARD:—*Elsie's* (71A Mt. Auburn, Cambridge, MA). Elsie's is to Harvard what White Castle is to college students elsewhere: the traditional way to cure a late-night/late-hour food fix. The Elsie burger and a slew of sandwiches are featured—the roast beef and the Fresser's Dream being the most popular—but don't bother to agonize over the long menu, since they all tend to taste the same. Still, they're filling, sloppy, and, before you know it, addicting. You'll even grow to like the Day-Glo green sawdust on the floor. Because, like Elsie's, it's there.

8.–UNIVERSITY OF SOUTHERN CALIFORNIA:—*Tommy's* (2575 Beverly Blvd., Los Angeles). Students at SC have a standing joke about Tommy's: If you get so drunk you forgot where you ate the night before, if you ate at Tommy's, you'll remember the next morning. But students aren't the only ones who flock to this twenty-four-hour dive. On any night, the parking lot is jammed with nearly every human type, including an occasional bathrobed patient from nearby St. Vincent's Hospital. All because of the burgers, a tribute to great American grease and buried under a thick smothering of chili and onions to produce one of the greasiest, messiest, most classic pig-outs around. There aren't too many stands like this one left. Especially at 2:00 A.M.

9.–PENN STATE:—
The Creamery (on campus, State College, PA). It started when they had to do something with all that milk put out by the agriculture school's herd of 150 cows. And now it's tradition. Daily, chocolate-starved, butter-fat-deficient students flood in to get a (literally) fresh fix of what has been rated by industry experts as one of the best ice creams in the country. Definitely makes the cost of tuition seem worthwhile.

10.–TULANE UNIVERSITY:—*The Camellia Grill* (626 S. Carrollton, New Orleans, LA). See WHERE TO PIG OUT: The Top Ten.

BAKER'S DOZEN

A random sampling of some sweet treats, where you can not only have your cake, but eat it, too.

1.–BONTÉ (1316 Third Avenue, New York). That rare French bakery where everything tastes even better than it looks. The pastries are buttery, flaky, crispy, and light; the only regret is having to choose one of them over the other. The tarts—especially the raspberry, if available—are outstanding.

2.–SALLY BELL'S (708 W. Grace Street, Richmond, VA). A distinctively Southern bakery where they should charge for the smells, they're so good. Box lunches are a specialty, as are the delicious biscuits, Sally Lunn breads, and lemon chess pies. But the crowning glory is their cupcake, which is turned upside-down after baking, then iced all around the sides and across the top. They're available in devil's food cake with chocolate or mocha icing, and yellow cake with chocolate, caramel, lemon, strawberry, or orange icings. To die for.

3.–MICHEL RICHARD (310 S. Robertson Blvd., Los Angeles). Meringues, religieuses, napoleons, éclairs . . . There are so many excellent choices here you really can't go wrong. Still, opt for the opera—alternating layers of chocolate and mocha cream, sandwiched between almond biscuits soaked in espresso, and coated with a thick, hard chocolate; or try the auteuil, a thin sponge cake soaked in raspberry puree, topped with chocolate truffle, and dusted with cocoa powder.

4.–VENIERO'S (342 East 11 Street, New York). An amazing selection of Italian breads, cookies, torrone, and gelati. The pastries come in both miniature and large sizes, enabling you to sample the smaller version first and then hoard up on what you think is best. Great cannoli, deliciously drenched (but not soggy) baba au rhum, crusty sfogliatelle.

5.–THE SWEET SOIREE (4182 E. Virginia Avenue, Denver). Beyond the double glass doors leading to this gourmet catering operation lies a small retail outlet where the display cases come brimming and the breads, cakes, and pastries are the true picture of pretentious pigging. But wait—the prices are reasonable, and every day three or four different treats (along with a jar of cookies filled with thirteen varieties, each better than the next) are laid out in a wooden hutch so that customers can taste and sample (hoard and scarf) while they struggle to make up their minds. Pray that there's a long line ahead of you; the best thing that can happen to you here is to be kept waiting.

6.—ROSIE'S BAKERY (243 Hampshire, Cambridge, MA). On a scale of one to ten, this place weighs in big. One bite and you are hooked. So much so that you'll be willing to fight Boston rush-hour traffic for Rosie's chocolate layer cake or butterscotch Congo bars; for her Chocolate Orgasm (a three-inch brownie, sinfully moist and chewy), you'll tackle a snowstorm.

7.–WATERGATE PASTRY SHOP (2534 Virginia Avenue, N.W., Washington, D.C.). This chic bakery in the bottom level of the infamous office building offers a dazzling array of goodies and—surprise—one of the best pig-out deals around. For three dollars they will fill a box with assorted end slices from their top-of-the-line, just-baked cakes and gâteaux. The boxes go on sale at 9:30 A.M., so waddle over early.

8.–PIONEER BOULANGERIE BAKERY (2012 Main Street, Santa Monica). There's a Basque influence working here, but the baked goods have a decidedly American feel. Either way, folks, you've hit the jackpot in Food City. Everything is wonderful: echoes of what mother used to make (trust me). Don't miss the sourdough bread, the cinnamon rolls, the pecan pie,

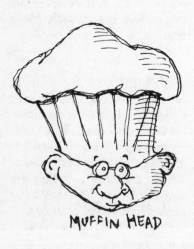

MUFFIN HEAD

the peanut-butter cookies, the lemon cake, the . . .

9.–LA MARQUISE (625 Chartres, New Orleans). This small, cramped patisserie offers a few seats, a view out onto the Quarter, and some of the best coffee and croissants around. Go in the afternoon, when it's less crowded, and you won't feel guilty about just you and your newspaper lingering at a window table for four. Whatever you do, try the "marquise"—a French pastry that's been given a definitive New Orleans touch: sponge cake, soaked in raspberry puree, is topped with mocha cream and pralines, and covered in a dark chocolate shell.

10.–THE CHEESE BOARD (1504 Shattuck, Berkeley). Some of the world's best—and most unusual—breads are baked in the kitchen at the back of this excellent cheese store. The baguettes alone deserve mention, but there are also terrific loaves of sourdough beer rye, buttermilk corn cheddar, Sunday bread (a honey-sweetened dough mixed with raisins, cinnamon, and walnuts), and challah. Discounts available for seniors and student piggers.

11.–MAISON ROBERT (3867 Peachtree Road, N.E., Atlanta).

This French-inspired bakery offers a little of everything, and has a larger tearoom in the back. While the cakes lack originality and are better to look at than to eat, the dinner rolls in particular are worth trying, with good texture and good flavor. But oddly enough, what really stands out here are the chocolate caramels, part of the limited candy selection buried away in an off-to-the-side display. A dark (chocolate) chewy center is covered with a layer of creamy milk chocolate, then rolled in raw sugar, giving it added sweetness, sparkle, and bite. A delightful contrast of textures; for chocoholics, they're a must.

12.–AMIGHETTI BAKERY (5141 Wilson, St. Louis). The best thing that this St. Louis institution bakes is a great Italian bread. It's also the only thing. A lackluster achievement, perhaps, but it's what they do with this loaf that keeps piggers coming back: "The Amighetti Special"—a sandwich ("often imitated, never duplicated") composed of layers of salami, cold beef, turkey, ham, mortadella, cheese, onions, hot peppers, lettuce, and tomato. Add some mustard, a little mayo, and it comes highly recommended. . . . The bread is also used to make another Amighetti favorite, the Salsiccia Pinwheel. Dough is ladled with a mixture of tomato sauce, sausage, onions, peppers, and olives, then rolled (in the manner of a log cake), baked, and sold either whole or by the slice. If you buy a slice, it's best to do so when it is fresh out of the oven; otherwise, if they warm it in the microwave, it tends to come out gummy.

13.–THE EROTIC BAKER (117 Christopher Street; plus additional locations, New York). If I knew you were coming, I'd have baked a cake. This is the place where custom-made cakes were first baked and iced to look like a few of the more interesting parts of the human anatomy. They get mentioned because of their originality. For their novelty. God only knows how they taste.

"I'LL GLADLY PAY YOU TUESDAY FOR A HAMBURGER TODAY"

If there is one food that is quintessentially piggy, it is the burger—a handful of meat, flung on a grill, smothered with mustard or ketchup, and nestled inside of a bun. Few other tastes are quite as fulfilling, or as sought-after, especially when accompanied by the cool contrast of a shake and the salt of some fries. And while you are scarfing down all that beautifully charred grease, you can even convince yourself that it is good for you. Hey, it's protein, isn't it?

Oddly, no documentation exists as to when the burger, as we know it, first got started. Some purists claim it was born at the St. Louis World's Fair of 1904, while others insist that credit should go to New Haven, Connecticut, lunch-counter-owner Louis Lassen. Whatever the case, one thing we do know is that the pigger who gave ground beef its initial push was J. H. Salisbury, an English physician who prescribed eating it three times a day. The taste caught on, and in America piggers nicknamed the meat "hamburger," after the German city, Hamburg, where the process of grinding steaks originated.

There are several schools of hamburger eaters, and whether a particular burger can be called "good" depends, of course, on which type of pigger is doing the talking. But basically, all burgers can be classified into one of two categories.

BURGERBURGERS. These are the thinner burgers, the lightweights, with less meat than bun, but still top-grade and delicious. These are the ones most "like they used to make," the old-fashioned kind they served at the drive-in, the drugstore, the malt shop, or the diner. Burgerburgers have a classic taste; they can be plump, but they are *never* fat.

BIGGERBURGERS. The most recent eating trend, the new burger on the block, the modern-day burger standard. These are the gourmet burgers, the thicker burgers, the fat boys who weigh in at at least a third of a pound. It is important to note that while all gourmet burgers are biggerburgers, not all biggerburgers are gourmet. All do, however, subscribe to the theory that enough is rarely enough.

Experience has shown that the most dependably good burgers fall somewhere in between; thick enough that the meat isn't overpowered by the bun or what's on it, and thin enough that you can lose yourself in it but still remain in charge. And while pigging preferences are obviously influenced by the pigger's mood at the moment, in the end, what makes a burger truly great is simply the combination of fresh meat on the right grill: that wonderful fusion of flavor and grease which is the very heart and soul of perfect pigging.

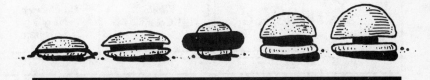

A CITY–BY–CITY GUIDE
TO BURGERS (AND FRIES AND SHAKES)

	Day 1	Day 2
LOS ANGELES *	*Fat Burger* 450 South La Cienga Blvd.	*Cassell's* 3300 W. 6th Street
NEW YORK **	*Waverly and Waverly* 153 Waverly Place	*Broome St. Bar* 363 West Broadway
CHICAGO	*Billy Goat Tavern* 430 N. Michigan	*R. J. Grunt's* 2056 Lincoln Park West
DALLAS	*Dunston's* 8526 Harry Hines Blvd.	*Snuffer's* 3526 Greenville
DETROIT	*Nemo's* 1384 Michigan Avenue	*Woodbridge Tavern* 289 St. Aubin
HOUSTON	*Roznovsky's* 5719 Feagan	*Fuddrucker's* 3100 Chimney Rock
SAN FRANCISCO	*Wim's* 141 Columbus	*Hamburger Mary's* 1582 Folsom

***Tommy's,** 2575 Beverly Blvd. (See p. 52.)
****The Burger Joint,** 2175 Broadway (See p. 53.)

A comprehensive look at some of the country's better burger towns, where it is possible to delight in not only a great burger, but a different burger, six days of the week. (*Six* days? Well, even He had to rest on the seventh.)

Day 3	Day 4	Day 5	Day 6
The Apple Pan 10801 W. Pico Blvd.	*Hampton's* 1342 N. Highland	*Hard Rock Cafe* 8600 Beverly Blvd.	*Sunset Grill* 7439 W. Sunset Blvd.
Empire Diner 210 Tenth Avenue	*J.G. Melon/J.G. Melon West* 1291 Third Avenue; 340 Amsterdam Avenue	*Moondance Diner* 80 Avenue of the Americas	*Jackson Hole Wyoming* 1633 Second Avenue
Red's Place 2200 W. Cermak	*Topnotch Burger* 1822 W. 95th	*Little John's* 210 W. Kinzie	*Charlie Beinlich* Skokie Highway
Kincaid's 4901 Camp Bowie, Fort Worth	*Stoneleigh P.* 2926 Maple	*Chili's* 7567 Greenville	*Lightfoot's* 221 S. Corinth, Oak Cliff
Monty's Grill 1120 N. Woodward Avenue, Royal Oak	*Lafayette Coney Island* 118 W. Lafayette	*Checker Bar and Grill* 124 Cadillac Square	*Fleetwood Diner* 300 S. Ashley, Ann Arbor
Otto's 1502 Memorial	*Old Bayou Inn* 216 Heights Blvd.	*Bellaire Broiler Burger* 5216 Bellaire Blvd.	*James' Restaurant* 6818 Chetwood
Bill's Place 2315 Clement	*Fat Apple's* 1346 Grove, Berkeley	*Original Joe's* 144 Taylor	

A CITY–BY–CITY GUIDE TO BURGERS (AND FRIES AND SHAKES)

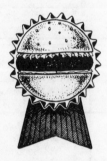

LOS ANGELES*

Fat Burger, 450 S. La Cienega Blvd.; plus other locations. Billed as "the last great hamburger stand," and they may be right. The double fatburger, with bacon and cheese, is unequaled, the king of the fast-food breed—satisfying and messy, perfectly seasoned, with just the right hit of grease. Open twenty-four hours. A great R & B jukebox, too.

Cassell's, 3300 W. 6th Street. The meat is ground daily and the burgers are out of this world; no doubt one of the best you're likely to find. Add to that homemade mayonnaise, ketchup, mustard, and dressings, along with garnishes, cottage cheese, fruit, and potato salad from a take-all-you-want buffet. No shakes, but homemade lemonade. Lunches only.

The Apple Pan, 10801 W. Pico Blvd. A horseshoe-shaped counter serving not one, but two, of the tastiest burgers around. (See WHERE TO PIG OUT: The Top Ten.)

Hampton's, 1342 N. Highland; plus second location. "A balanced meal is a hamburger in each hand," though the burgers here are so big you might be hard-pressed to handle even one. Still, they're terrific, especially the gourmet "Slam Dunkburger," topped with Dijon mustard and sour-plum jam.

Hard Rock Cafe, 8600 Beverly Blvd. An offshoot of the famed London joint, you'll recognize this one by the '59 Cadillac crashing into the roof. Loud, campy, with blaring rock music, and waitresses dressed in fifties starched white uniforms. When cooked right, burgers are excellent, about as good as they can get. Fries are also a plus: thin, crisp, and brown, with the skins still on. Great shakes, but they come in an old-fashioned glass that's much too small.

Sunset Grill, 7439 W. Sunset Blvd. A raffish, delightful dive (with an outside counter that practically sits on the street), serving up a pigging standard: a good *cheap* burger cooked on a greasy grill and smothered in Velveeta cheese. A place to hit only when the mood is right, but when it's right, nothing's better.

---

*__Tommy's,__ 2575 Beverly Blvd. Any day of the week, but only at 2:00 A.M. (See WHERE TO PIG OUT: The Big Ten/University of Southern California.)

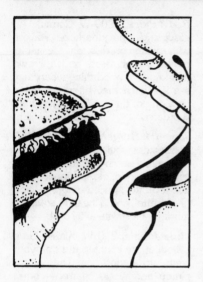

NEW YORK*

Waverly and Waverly, 153 Waverly Place (between Avenue of the Americas and Seventh Avenue). The place is new, but from the old-fashioned soda fountain with the mirrored-back bar to the thirties Wurlitzer jukebox, it looks like a set straight out of *Ozzie & Harriet*. A *real* burger, too, nothing gimmicky or oversophisticated. Milk shakes are served in their stainless-steel containers, wonderfully thick and big enough for two.

Broome St. Bar, 363 West Broadway. Good size, good quality and charcoaled to boot (though it's hard for a serious pigger not to laugh at the pita-bread bun).

Empire Diner, 210 Tenth Avenue (between 22nd and 23rd streets).

Perfectly charred, and when you say "rare," they actually know how to do it. So what if it comes with a garnish of seedless grapes? The epitome of the upscale-burger breed.

J.G. Melon/J.G. Melon West, 1291 Third Avenue; 340 Amsterdam Avenue. Plump and juicy, with good flavor. Definitely a "pub" burger: more of a snack than a meal, but still, too often underrated.

Moondance Diner, 80 Avenue of the Americas (at Grand). A true-blue diner serves a true-blue burger with true-blue-burger taste. The only problem is that it comes with true-blue *potato skins*. They're good, but a burger this traditional demands fries, so ask for a substitution. In the meantime, pull up a stool and drown your troubles in a serious chocolate shake.

Jackson Hole Wyoming, 1633 Second Avenue (at 85th). A local favorite (if only it were char-broiled instead of grilled). Still, it's huge and generously topped, to the point of perfect sloppiness. Fries are good, but avoid the onion rings.

---

*__*The Burger Joint,__* 2175 Broadway; 1489 Second Avenue. Quality and quantity. (See HOW TO PIG OUT: How to Pig Out When There's Nothing in the House/The Telephone.)

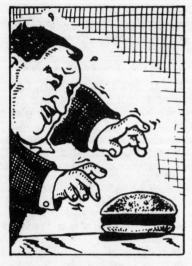

CHICAGO

Billy Goat Tavern, 430 N. Michigan. "Cheeseburger, cheeseburger, cheeseburger . . ." Hidden beneath Michigan Avenue near the Chicago Tribune building, this hole-in-the-wall grill is one of the most celebrated burger joints around, having served as the inspiration for the infamous *Saturday Night Live* sketch. The burgers are just what you'd expect—all very tasty and perfectly greasy. Needless to say, they don't serve fries. But order them anyway.

R.J. Grunt's, 2056 Lincoln Park West. The kind of place you love to hate and end up liking anyway; just ignore the cutesy menu and remember what you're here for: a top-of-the-line, gourmet burger, properly cooked and among the finest. Steak fries, too—some thick, some thin, all delicious.

Red's Place, 2200 W. Cermak. An easygoing, neighborhood tavern with plates of dills on the table, motherly waitresses, and a crowd that knows a good thing when they see it. Which they often do, every time one of the terrific burgers here is ordered.

Topnotch Burger, 1822 W. 95th. A nondescript sixties counter-and-tables setting serving an authentic burger with a good, old-fashioned taste. Top it off with grilled onions, a glob of ketchup, and a healthy squirt of mustard. Nostalgia at its best.

Little John's, 210 W. Kinzie. Grab a stool at the counter and sink your teeth into a good one. The patty—plump and nicely charred—comes on black bread that complements but doesn't overpower. Tell them rare and they'll listen.

Charlie Beinlich, Skokie Highway (between Dundee and Lake Cook), Northbrook. The best of the burgs in the burbs; meaty, flavorful, and cooked to perfection.

DALLAS

Dunston's, 8526 Harry Hines Blvd.; plus other locations. An extraordinarily well-executed burger that not only holds its own but, at just under two bucks, could be the best burger buy for your money. They butter and toast the bun as well as grill the patty, right along with the steaks, over mesquite. Score two points for style.

Snuffer's, 3526 Greenville. A small restaurant/bar where at first glance you might expect the food to be as commonplace as the natural-oak decor. Wrong. The limited twelve-item menu features a huge, mouth-watering burger served on a poppy-seed bun with all the right ingredients; the homemade fries (see WHERE TO PIG OUT: The Best of the Rest/Best French Fries) will surpass your wildest expectations.

Kincaid's, 4901 Camp Bowie, Fort Worth. Actually a local grocery store, where burgers are sold from behind the meat counter. And they are excellent. Thick, juicy, and eight ounces of savory proof that the thirty-mile drive from Dallas to Fort Worth is more than a pigging alternative, it's a must.

Stoneleigh P., 2926 Maple. A Dallas favorite—and onetime pharmacy—the food (and drink) here is as good as hanging out. The burgers are top of the line, with a touch of imagination: provolone cheese and pumpernickel bread. There's even a magazine stand for free reading while you eat. Current issues, too.

Chili's, 7567 Greenville; plus other locations, including Houston, San Antonio, Atlanta, Denver, and San Jose. There is a slew of Chili's now, but the burgers remain a prime example of the good things that can come from a chain restaurant. High quality, thick, and perfectly cooked—and available in a variety of incarnations. Don't miss the chili. And don't miss the fries, either—

skinny, golden brown, and home-made.

Lightfoot's, 221 S. Corinth, Oak Cliff. The curb service has been discontinued, the hours are inconsistent (Mon.-Wed.-Fri.-Sat. after 1:00 P.M.) and the burgers, while good, are on the thin side, with a little too much bun for the beef. But what owner Rufus Lightfoot does right—besides play a mean game of pinball—is blend up a terrific shake, so thick and creamy that, as they say in the commercial, you might have to eat it with a spoon.

DETROIT

Nemo's, 1384 Michigan Avenue. There are other locations, too, but none quite like the first, a neighborhood bar just down the road from the ball park. The burger grill in the back room fixes up a great one: juicy, thick, and flavorful.

Woodbridge Tavern, 289 St. Aubin. It's a trendy, bar-hopping crowd, but it's also a damn fine burger—nicely charred, beautifully garnished, with the best of burger tastes. Bite for bite, probably the best in town.

Monty's Grill, 1120 N. Woodward Avenue, Royal Oak. A down-home Mom-and-Pop operation housed at a local motel, offering a simple, basic burger, reliably good, and topped with the tastiest smoked bacon around. No frills, no fuss; well worth a visit.

Lafayette Coney Island, 118 W. Lafayette. The downtown dive that's responsible for a Detroit pigging standard: a steamed hot-dog roll filled with browned ground beef and finished off with chopped onions, mustard, and chili. An eye-opening change of pace.

Checker Bar and Grill, 124 Cadillac Square. Although the place has expanded and remodeled—and lost a great deal of its original hole-in-the-wall charm—it still puts out a mountain of a burger well worth your while. The toasty sesame seed bun is an added plus.

Fleetwood Diner, 300 S. Ashley, Ann Arbor. Noted for their infamous "Chili Size" special: one cheeseburger, an order of fries, and the whole shebang buried under a layer of prize-winning homemade chili. For those who have done it all, one of pigging's more daring experiences. (The burger good on its own, by the way.)

HOUSTON

Roznovsky's, 5719 Feagan. This used to be a corner grocery store, and it still looks like a corner grocery store. But they quit selling groceries because the burger business got too good. And deservedly so. A basic burger with everything to make it one of the best.

Fuddrucker's, 3100 Chimney Rock. A twenty-first-century hamburger stand. A slick, white-tiled self-service restaurant where the beef is ground fresh (right in front of you), comes thick (eight-ounce patties), is cooked to order, and served on an oversized homemade bun. Dress it yourself with an array of fresh garnishes from multiple trays and tables of produce. Sure, the place reeks of gimmicks, but that aside, this could be the burger of your dreams.

Otto's, 5502 Memorial. This longtime favorite of the downtown lunch bunch became famous for its barbecue, but in a separate building turns out burgers that surpass everything else on the menu. Good taste, slightly messy, one of the top in town.

Old Bayou Inn, 216 Heights Blvd. A fast-paced, college-type hangout where the burgers are big, the beer is cold, and the chips are homemade.

Bellaire Broiler Burger, 5216 Bellaire Blvd. They couldn't have named this place better if they tried. No fancy hoopla—just a good burger, charcoal broiled over an open flame.

James' Restaurant, 6818 Chetwood. This one has a boring, prefabricated look, but the burgers taste anything but. And the fries are exceptional—cut fresh, fried crisp, and left in their skins.

SAN FRANCISCO

Wim's, 141 Columbus. A sixties lunch counter lined with individual table-top jukeboxes, this is the place to eat your burger fantasies: freshly ground meat, deliciously charred, and available with—get this—*real* French fries, and double-thick shakes in their stainless-steel containers. (The daily specials are just that—from pork chops to pasta to coq au vin. Check them out.) Breakfast and lunch only.

Hamburger Mary's, 1582 Folsom. Tucked away in a warehouse district, this eclectic eatery is bustling, combining an interesting mix of people with a fun, San Francisco feeling. Baby bottles double as cream dispensers; the burgers are truly good, served on whole wheat bread, topped with tomato, onions, sprouts, and special sauces—a biggerburger that's neither pampered nor overworried.

Bill's Place, 2315 Clement; plus second location. Everything you want in a burger and more. No fancy frills, just excellent beef (ground daily), fresh condiments (ruby-red tomatoes, a heaping of grilled onions), and superb taste. Mustard and ketchup come in old-fashioned squirt bottles; waitresses are worth their salt.

Fat Apple's, 1346 Grove, Berkeley. Top-quality beef is ground on the premises, hand-patted, and cooked to order. Served on a white or whole wheat bun, and topped with a mound of grated cheese, this is wonderful and sloppy at its best. The homemade pies are an added delight (see WHERE TO PIG OUT: The Best of the Rest/Best Apple Pie); make sure you try the fresh raspberry when in season. . . .

Original Joe's, 144 Taylor. An Italian restaurant might seem the last place you would expect to find a great burger, but then, this is no ordinary burger, either. It's a San Francisco institution, a whopping three-quarters of a pound, grilled with a touch of onion and an assortment of spices for flavoring. The roll is a hollowed-out loaf of sourdough French bread. Massive, thick, and juicy, there's enough here for tomorrow night's dinner as well, plus leftovers.

In your quest for the best, if the only direct flight has a three-hour layover in Kansas City, or if the snow leaves you stranded in Milwaukee, have no fear, great pigging is here: **Solly's** (4620 N. Port Washington Road, Milwaukee) offers the tops in the "wonderful and greasy" burger tradition; **Winstead's** (101 Brush Creek, Kansas City) serves up double and triple steakburgers, along with their exclusive chocolate spoon malt, proving that drive-ins of old have not become extinct.

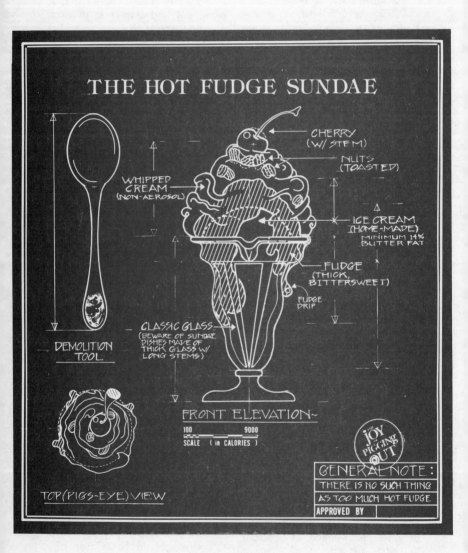

THE HOT FUDGE SUNDAE

DEMOLITION TOOL

WHIPPED CREAM (NON-AEROSOL)

CHERRY (W/ STEM)

NUTS (TOASTED)

ICE CREAM (HOME-MADE) MINIMUM 14% BUTTER FAT

FUDGE (THICK, BITTERSWEET)

FUDGE DRIP

CLASSIC GLASS (BEWARE OF SUNDAE DISHES MADE OF THICK GLASS W/ LONG STEMS)

FRONT ELEVATION~

100   9000
SCALE (in CALORIES)

THE JOY PIGGING OUT

GENERAL NOTE:
THERE IS NO SUCH THING
AS TOO MUCH HOT FUDGE

APPROVED BY

TOP (PIGS-EYE) VIEW

LA CRÈME DE LA CREAM

The hard, cold facts . . .

Fact: In the thirteenth century, Marco Polo returned from his voyage to the Orient carrying a recipe for a frozen dessert made with ice and milk.

Fact: In the winter of 1794, Beethoven lived in fear, not of being unable to finish his symphony, but that the unseasonably mild Vienna weather would not leave enough ice for the coming summer to make an ample supply of ice cream.

Fact: In the 1920s, immigrants arriving at Ellis Island were served ice cream as part of their first American meal; baffled, many attempted to spread it on their bread.

Fact: During World War II, the navy built a million-dollar "floating ice-cream parlor" to supply the wantful troops in the Pacific and help boost sailor morale.

Fact: Before the days of Vietnam protests, 1,500 Yale students rioted for hours when police forced a Humpty-Dumpty ice-cream cart to leave the campus.

Fact is everybody screams for it, yet nobody ever agrees on which is the absolute best. Why bother? Since most premium ice creams are hometown specialties—or distributed only in a limited area—what's tops in Topeka probably isn't even available in Atlanta. So for jet-setting piggers, as well as those who will go anywhere to get their licks, here is a guide to *the best* ice cream in the country, depending, of course, on where you are when you want it. . . .

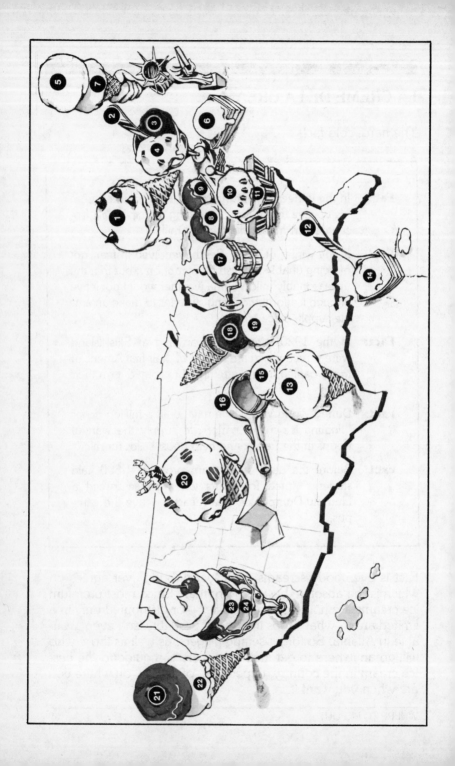

1. **Ben & Jerry's,** 169 Cherry, Burlington, VT.
Why: Black raspberry, Heath Bar crunch, mint Oreo; their chocolate-chip flavors include the whole morsel, not just a chip of the whole morsel; on a good day, lucky customers get to lick the dasher when a fresh batch is finished.

2. **Steve's,** 191 Elm, Somerville, MA.
Why: Chocolate cinnamon raisin; for revolutionizing ice-cream eating practices by introducing the idea of mix-ins—the flavor of your choice is thrown onto a slab and into it is carefully kneaded such varied goodies as M & M's, mixed nuts, butterscotch chips, crumbled Oreos, or ground-up Reese's Peanut Butter Cups.

3. **Emack & Bolio's,** 1310 Massachusetts Avenue, Cambridge, MA.
Why: As boring as it sounds, the vanilla—pure, sweet, and creamy—and any other flavor using it, particularly the Oreo.

4. **Steve Herrell's Ice Cream,** 150 Main, Northampton, MA.
Why: This is Steve—yes, *that* Steve—who founded the legendary aforementioned Steve's in Boston. After he sold the original place in 1977, he went west. About 100 miles west, where he opened a second shop. Every bit as good as, if not better than, the first.

5. **Pat Mitchell's,** 434 E. Main, Endicott, NY.
Why: The environment (buy a cone and eat it on the wall of the cemetery next door); the chocolate chips (milk chocolate and hand-chopped from an imported ten-pound candy bar); they deliver.

6. **Robert's,** 660 North Highway, Southampton, NY.
Why: Originality; chocolate peanut-butter cup; fresh peach; for being the first to introduce an Oreo flavor.

7. **Häagen-Dazs,** available nationwide, but a born and bred New Yorker.
Why: For going where no other chain had dared to go—to 16 percent butterfat and, damn the costs, to the very best ingredients, with no stabilizers, no preservatives, no corn syrup, and no ice milk; the chocolate chocolate chip, the coffee chip, the rum raisin . . .

8. **Bassett's,** Reading Terminal, Philadelphia, PA.
Why: Longevity; Irish coffee; 18 percent butterfat.

9. **Hilary's,** 437 South Street, Philadelphia, PA.
Why: Best topping selection (thirty-two in all, including eight nuts, six fruits, two kinds of brownies); s'mores (chocolate ice cream with graham crackers and marshmallow); superb hot fudge.

10. **Inside Scoop,** 1134 19th Street, N.W., Washington, D.C.

(Continued)

Why: Chocolate Amaretto, sweet cream; new flavors are developed from a customer suggestion list that hangs by the door; "Happy Hour" every Friday, 3:00–6:00 P.M.: two scoops for the price of one on all flavors made with rum or liqueur.

11. **Bob's Famous,** 236 Massachusetts Avenue, Washington, D.C.
Why: Kahlúa, orange chocolate chocolate-chip, coffee Oreo; for recognizing life's priorities, in that famous Bob gave up the practice of law to devote himself to making great ice cream.

12. **Steve's Homemade Ice Cream,** 1172 Peachtree, Atlanta, GA.
(No relation to Steve's in Boston—or Steve Herrell's in Northampton—but definitely patterned after their success.)
Why: Cinnamon (even better when served atop a piece of apple pie from the nearby Pleasant Peasant, 555 Peachtree); the ice-cream "omelets."

13. **Neal's,** 2826 Kirby, Houston, TX.
Why: Bananas Foster (banana ice cream with caramelized bananas swirled in it); tré scalini (a dark chocolate ice cream made with unprocessed chocolate liquor); the imported cones from Denmark.

14. **Angelo Brocato,** 214 N. Carrollton, New Orleans, LA.
Why: The Italian ices, particularly the lemon; spumone, cassata (spumone with cake), terrancino (vanilla, almond,

and cinnamon), Italian chocolate (chocolate, almond, and cinnamon).

15. **Miss Hulling's Creamery,** 7022 Clayton Avenue, St. Louis, MO.
Why: The best soft-serve ice cream—chocolate and vanilla, (so ask for a half-and-half); the freezer selection—Marmadukes (soft ice cream dipped in chocolate and on a stick), Monkey Sticks (frozen bananas dipped in chocolate), and Mr. Frisbees (a soft-ice-cream ice-cream sandwich).

16. **Crown Candy Kitchen,** 1401 St. Louis Avenue, St. Louis, MO.
Why: A genuine ice-cream parlor, complete with soda fountain, homemade chocolates, and table service; hot fudge that, when it cools, becomes a rich, partly chewy, partly brittle candy; chocolate malts that can be ordered with bits of banana; the turtle sundae.

17. **Graeter's,** numerous locations, Cincinnati, OH.
Why: Lots of cream, an incredibly fresh taste; any "chip" flavor, all made "the French pot way"—the chocolate is poured in as a liquid, hardening, as the ice cream is being cranked, into melt-in-your-mouth chunks.

18. **Ting-a-Ling,** 42 W. Division Street, Chicago, IL.
Why: They don't make them like this anymore: a small fountain, worn leather booths, and a slightly dusty feel; the coffee ice cream with hot fudge (bit-

tersweet and good—if only there were more of it); real whipped cream.

19. **Dove's Candies,** 6000 South Pulaski Road, Chicago, IL.
Why: The hand-dipped ice-cream bars (the ice cream *could* use a fuller flavor, but one bite into the quarter-inch-thick chocolate coating and you'll forget about such minor technicalities).

20. **Lickety Split,** 2031 E. 13th Avenue, Denver, CO.
Why: Cheesman Park (cheese cake ice cream with a strawberry marble running through it), brandy banana nut (with English walnuts); they'll actually custom-make any flavor to suit your pigging needs.

21. **Gelato Classico,** numerous locations, San Francisco, CA.
Why: Dense and rich, with a unique "pully" quality; even in a small cup you can get two flavors at once; coppa mista (chocolate, vanilla, pistachio, and almond) and the possible dark chocolate and peanut-butter combination.

22. **Double Rainbow,** 407 Castro; plus other locations, San Francisco, CA.
Why: The winner of the first Great American Ice Cream Lick-Off held in Philadelphia in 1982. (Note: The vanilla is good, as is the white pistachio, but due to the ultra-high butterfat content, some flavors tend to get too chewy. A warning: Taste first.)

23. **Robin Rose Ice Cream,** 215 Rose Avenue, Venice, CA.

Why: Chic and trendy, an inordinately high liquor content ("the over-21 ice cream"); Apple A la mode, raspberry chocolate truffle (chocolate ice cream, raspberry Chambord liqueur and chunks of wonderous chocolate truffles); the neon list-of-flavors sign.

24. **C. C. Brown's,** 7007 Hollywood Blvd., Hollywood, CA.
Why: An old-fashioned sundae in an old-fashioned setting—complete with high-backed mahogany booths and family portraits; hot fudge, as perfect as it gets, served on the side and in a creamer-sized porcelain pitcher you get to lick clean when you are finished; and almonds, not only toasted but salted. (A warning: For the size, expensive.)

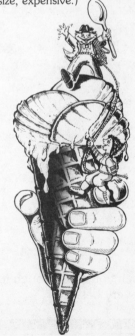

THE COOKIE
HALL OF FAME*

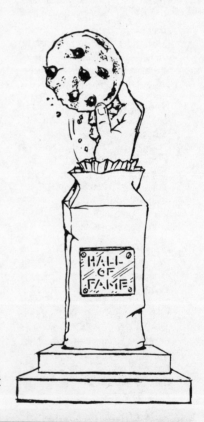

When you care enough to eat
the very best.

DAVID'S CHOCOLATE CHUNK, *David's Cookies* (1018 Second Avenue, New York; plus selected locations nationwide). The Rolls-Royce of the chocolate-chip cookie world. Soft, warm, moist, with pure butter, and chips so big they had to call them chunks. Which they are—nonuniform, cut-up pieces of Lindt chocolate (that ooze in the mouth) in proportions to boggle the mind of even the most jaded pigger. The other variations—especially the "peanut-butter chocolate chunk," and even the Lindtless "raisin oatmeal"—also excel.

FRANGO MINT COOKIES, *Marshall Field stores* (Chicago; additional locations in Houston, Dallas). A thin, crisp cookie daintily loaded with bits of meltingly delicious mint chocolate to produce a distinctive, sophisticated taste. Perfect for after dinner or a secret midnight rendezvous.

SESAME SEED COOKIE, *The Missouri Bakery* (2027 Edward Street, St. Louis). Light, airy, crunchy, covered in a sea of sesame seeds, and good enough to turn a cup of tea into an afternoon pig-out.

GINGER COOKIE, *Betsy's Place* (144 E. 74th Street, New York). Textured and chewy, with just the right snap to its flavor, and a faint sprinkling of sugar across the top for added bite.

BUTTERSCOTCH COOKIE, *Pioneer Boulangerie Bakery* (2012 Main Street, Santa Monica). Tiny pieces of hard butterscotch surrounded by a crumbly, buttery cookie that melts in your mouth.

MILANO (Pepperidge Farm); MYSTIC MINT (Nabisco). The top of the line of the prepackaged, nationally distributed brands. Both offer uniquely wonderful combinations of chocolate and cookie. But more important, they are reliable, like old friends.

---

*Members were selected not only on the basis of their good taste, but on their originality and upholding of century-old baking traditions. Nominations for new members are currently being accepted. All submissions become the property of the author of this book, who regrets that samples cannot be returned.

THE SANDWICH
HALL OF FAME

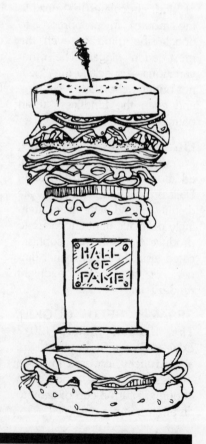

Breadwinners, all . . .

FERDI SPECIAL, *Mother's* (401 Poydras, New Orleans, LA). The epitome—the best—of the New Orleans Poor Boys. A wondrously oversized sandwich of baked ham and roast beef (thickly cut, freshly carved) covered with stewed-beef drippings from yesterday's leftovers (ah, the juice!), and slathered with lettuce, mayonnaise, and two mustards. All on an excellent French roll. One bite is worth a thousand words. And good thing . . . you won't want to stop eating long enough to talk.

CHEESESTEAK, *Jim's Steaks* (400 South Street; 431 N. 62nd Street, Philadelphia, PA). The genuine Philadelphia sandwich from—where else?—the city that made it famous. Grilled, paper-thin slices of steak are spooned into a long Italian roll along with molten cheese (real cheese, none of this processed-spread stuff, thank you), and a variety of mushroom, pepper, onion, and sauce toppings. A wonderfully greasy blur of flavors and tastes.

THE ORIGINAL SLOPPY JOE, *Town Hall Delicatessen* (18 S. Orange Avenue, South Orange, NJ). No hamburger meat in tomato sauce here. Rather, what you get is an original version of an old deli standard, the combination sandwich. And it's outstanding. A loaf of rye bread is cut lengthwise, into long, ultra-thin slices, after which the crusts are trimmed to give each piece a rectangular shape. The slices are then smeared with coleslaw and Thousand Island dressing and stacked vertically, with alternating layers of turkey, rare roast beef, and Swiss cheese. When this multilevel masterpiece is finally assembled, it is cut into square pieces, each looking like some sort of delicatessen petit four. Delicious.

SLICED-BEEF SANDWICH, *Sonny Bryan's* (2202 Inwood Road, Dallas, TX). Honest-to-goodness Texas barbecue—hickory-smoked brisket of beef—is trimmed of fat, sliced to order, and piled high and thick on a white-bread bun. The meat is distractingly juicy on its own, but add the sauce (from the individualized glass shaker bottles on the side) and pigging out reaches a level of bliss heretofore only dreamed of.

BARBECUE, Bill's Barbecue (5805 Broad Street, Richmond, VA). Forget Washington, Jefferson, and Robert E. Lee. To piggers from Virginia and North Carolina, *this* is the South's favorite son: finely minced pork, mixed with a tangy hot sauce, and topped with chopped coleslaw. A bit of heaven on a bun.

MUFFULETTA, The Central Grocery (923 Decatur, New Orleans, LA). A round loaf of Italian bread—baked by the United Bakery and great on its own—is made even better with layered, top-of-the-line Genoa salami, Holland ham, mortadella, Swiss cheese, and a marinated olive salad. Despite its ethnic name, this New Orleans classic is unheard-of anywhere in Italy. If they only knew what they were missing.

CUBAN SANDWICH, Latin American Cafeteria (2940 SW 22 Street, Miami, FL). Ham, pork, and Swiss cheese, with mustard and pickles, stacked on a long roll and grilled to a melted crisp. Also called the "midnight special"—which it is, twenty-four hours a day.

ITALIAN BEEF, Al's Bar-B-Q (1079 W. Taylor Street, Chicago, IL). In Chicago, Italian beef is as common as wind; highly seasoned meat is cooked slowly and sliced thin, then soaked in a gravy that has been flavored with oregano, black pepper, and garlic, and served with sweet and hot peppers on a skinny Italian loaf. A juicy, oily eye-opener, so spicy that it will make your lips, your mouth, and every taste bud tingle.

CHINESE ROAST PORK, The Subway (4037 Radford, Studio City, CA). On garlic bread, with plum sauce and hot mustard. If you think it *sounds* good, wait until you taste it. An inspired combination.

GRINDER (HOUSE SPECIAL), Mario's (4747 Wyandotte, Kansas City, MO). A hero of a sandwich. The tip of an individual-sized Italian loaf is cut off, about one and a half inches from the end, and the bread in the middle is scooped out. Next, into the hollowed crust are stuffed either sausages or meatballs (both are terrific) along with mozarella cheese, oregano, and the tomato-based sauce in which the meats were cooked. After that, the cut-off end is put back over the opened portion—but turned around, to function like a plug—and the sealed loaf is wrapped in foil, baked in the oven, and served. All very upper crust.

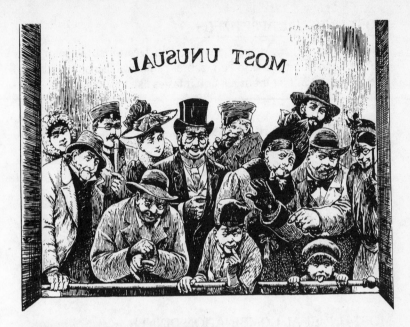

MOST UNUSUAL HAMBURGER

Hippo Hamburgers (Van Ness at Pacific Avenue, San Francisco, CA). The Hamburger Sundae. A charcoal-broiled six-ounce patty, smothered with vanilla ice cream and topped with sliced pickles, hot fudge, chopped nuts, and a maraschino cherry.

MOST UNUSUAL HOT DOG

Danny's Dogs (7450 Santa Monica Blvd., Los Angeles, CA). Danny's Oki (for Okinawa) Dog. It's actually two hot dogs, along with pastrami, chili, and cheese, wrapped in a flour tortilla.

MOST UNUSUAL ICE CREAM FLAVOR

Toscanini's (899 Main Street, Cambridge, MA).* Fig.

---

*Toscanini's also wins points for having the most original flavor. While every other homemade ice cream shop is dishing out "Oreo," Toscanini's offers "Hydrox."

MOST UNUSUAL APPETIZERS

Adam's Rib (40 S. Main, Zionsville, IN). Deep-fried alligator and braised kangaroo tails. Also lion, zebra, camel, rattlesnake, and buffalo hump. (Don't let them tell you it tastes like chicken.)

MOST UNUSUAL CHOCOLATES

Bayard's (2329 Marlton Park, Cherry Hill, NJ). Chocolate-covered cheese-and-peanut-butter crackers. In either light or dark.

MOST UNUSUAL STREET VENDOR

LaCart Chevalean (Lexington Avenue, between 53rd and 54th, New York, NY). Horseburgers. Made with 100 percent lean horse-meat.

MOST UNUSUAL COMBINATION DINNER

Alfie's (3301 S. Shepherd, Houston, TX). Fried cod, egg roll, burrito, and fries—$2.99 (price subject to change without notice).

MOST UNUSUAL FAST–FOOD RESTAURANT

Hop-Scotch (Chauncey Hill Mall, West Lafayette, IN). Fried rabbit. By the bucket or on a bun. With your choice of sweet-and-sour or barbecue sauce.

MOST UNUSUAL RESTAURANT NAME

Salad Bar (Phoenix, AZ). It doesn't have one.

MOST UNUSUAL RESTAURANT THEME

The Magic Time Machine (5003 Beltline Road, Dallas, TX). Sensory overload. Don't be surprised if Superman or Mata Hari shows up to check your coat, seat you at your table, or ask to take your order. Each nook and cranny of this bustling restaurant is decorated in a different motif. Dine in the back of a school bus, Sherlock Holmes's library, a giant crayon box, or an island tiki hut. The soup and salad bar is actually a soup and salad *car,* housed in a red MG convertible. Oh, yeah, the steaks aren't bad, either.

MOST UNUSUAL FOOD FESTIVAL

The Great American Pig-Out (various locations nationwide; a traveling show held on selected Sundays throughout the year. Call (615) 847-8610 for details). Southern barbecue, stuffed sausage, and grilled hot dogs are served amid an environment of camel rides, skydiving pigs, and games with names like Ring-A-Redneck and Corn Cob Hobble. Male exotic dancers, too.

MOST UNUSUAL SAYING ON A RESTAURANT MENU

Vivian's Place (10968 Ventura Blvd., Studio City, CA). "All sandwiches are served on bread."

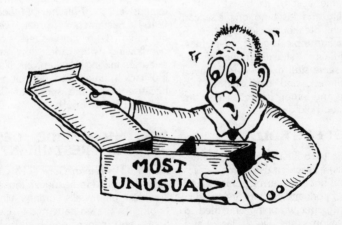

THE BEST OF THE REST

BEST TAKE-OUT CHICKEN

Chirping Chicken (350 Amsterdam at 77th, New York). Golden-brown and juicy, grilled over charcoals, and basted with garlic and lemon. Served with a nice twist: warmed pita bread and fresh tomato salsa. Sorry, Colonel.

BEST CHAIN RESTAURANT

Steak 'n Shake (locations in Florida, Georgia, Illinois, Indiana, Iowa, Kentucky, Missouri, Ohio, Tennessee). Try to ignore the fact that some of the restaurants have put in a salad bar and added to the original menu. So what if they don't have carhops anymore? This chain still offers the best of its breed, with a quality and taste no one else can match. Steakburgers (singles, doubles, and triples), good (crisp) fries, "tru-flavor" shakes (none of this soft-serve stuff excreted from metal machines), and old-fashioned orange and lemon freezes. These *are* the good old days.

BEST EGG ROLL

Matin (416 First Avenue N, Minneapolis). Black mushrooms, cellophane noodles, carrots, onions, and bits of pork and chicken are rolled in a rice-paper wrapping and fried to perfection: thin, light, lacy, and crisp. Served with a sweet, slightly spicy marinade. Available for take-out, but, alas, they don't deliver.

BEST PENNY CANDY SELECTION

Spicer's 5 & 10 (8817 Ladue Road, St. Louis). Penny candy is an anachronism, but Spicer's does sell three-cent candies, and every kind imaginable. Six rows, of four shelves each, are brimming with boxes of individually wrapped hard, soft, chewy, crunchy, gummy delights. . . . For a good selection of old-style penny candies that can't be bought individually but are weighed and sold by the pound, check out the candy counter at *Heaven* (10250 Santa Monica Blvd., Los Angeles). Heaven changes its stock most frequently, giving the best overall pick, but it's also the most expensive. . . . *Fletcher McLean* (2484 Sacramento Street, San Francisco) is a closet-sized store overflowing with candy jars and salesmen in long white aprons. It's a trip back in time, but a difficult one because hours are sporadic. Call first—(415) 567-8669.

BEST HOMEMADE DESSERTS IN A RESTAURANT

Ralph's American Cafe (143 Giralda, Miami). Home never looked like this: pink walls, orange vinyl booths, swirled-patterned tiled floors, and leopard-skin bar stools. Fresh flowers are placed on each table, but in Coke instead of the typical Perrier bottles. Dessert selections vary nightly—Innkeeper's Pie, chocolate-chip cake—but they're guaranteed to make you feel as good as the decor does. *Empire Diner* (210 Tenth Avenue, New York). The sleek black-and-chrome look, the live entertainment, and the candles on the counter are more upscale than your typical roadside diner, but the desserts, despite their fancy names (like "Espresso Cake" for devil's food cake with mocha icing), are the genuine thing.

BEST LEMONADE

Constant Lemonade (vendor, Kennedy Park, Miami). A frozen version, good in any form—from the first slushy slurp to the last melted-down drop.

BEST LIMEADE

Bill's Barbecue (5805 Broad Street, Richmond, VA). Squeezed by hand, right before your eyes; tart and tangy with the perfect hit of carbonation.

BEST FUDGE

Findley's Fabulous Fudge (1035 Geary Street, San Francisco). Made with whipping cream, using a blend of milk, semi-, and bittersweet chocolates, and a combination of white and brown sugars. The result is unbelievably smooth, rich, and creamy. In twelve terrific flavors.

BEST PIE (*when cut, would contain one slice of each of the following*):

APPLE: *Fat Apple's* (1346 Grove, Berkeley). One hundred percent American—no crumb topping, no raisins, no nuts—just chock-full of firm green apples, giving it a

sweet, tart taste. Served warm, with a scoop of vanilla or a chunk of sharp cheddar.

PECAN: *Camellia Grill* (626 S. Carrollton, New Orleans). A Southern favorite. Not too gritty, not too sweet, but with just the right consistency. Loaded with chopped pecans.

STRAWBERRY: *Reeve's Restaurant & Bakery* (1209 F Street, N.W., Washington, D.C.). Whole, luscious strawberries, without the overwhelming glaze, piled high in a flaky crust, and finished with a dollop of fresh whipped cream. Available year round here, two ways, either open-face or topped with crisscrossed strips of tender pastry.

BANANA CREAM: *The Apple Pan* (10801 W. Pico Blvd., Los Angeles). More bananas than custard, a heady layer of fresh whipped cream, and a crust that the French would envy. Perfect.

CHOCOLATE CREAM: *Bill's Barbecue* (5805 Broad Street, Richmond, Va.) An honest-to-goodness chocolate pie that doesn't taste like pudding or mousse. Dark and rich, in a good, thin crust.

ICE-CREAM PIE: Mile-High Ice-Cream Pie, *Cafe Pontchartrain* (Pontchartrain Hotel, 2031 St. Charles Avenue, New Orleans). A piecrust is filled with three layers of ice cream (one each of chocolate, vanilla, and peppermint), then topped with eight inches of meringue and a rich hot chocolate sauce.

BEST CHOCOLATE CAKE
(*like Mother used to make*)

Rumbuls (20 Christopher Street, New York). A delicious devil's food: dark, moist, and rich. Several variations daily; try the two-layer cake with raspberry frosting or the fudge iced version with a whipped-cream pocket in the center.

BEST CHOCOLATE CAKE
(*like Mother couldn't make*)

Cocolat (3324 Steiner Street, San Francisco). "Chocolate Decadence"—a perfect chocolate torte (sealed in a slick chocolate glaze) topped with a mountain of whipped cream, grated chocolate curls, and a raspberry puree. Good to the bitter-(sweet) end.

BEST OYSTER BAR

Felix's Restaurant (739 Iberville, New Orleans). This stand-up bar is overcrowded, unkempt, inexpensive, and a delight. Oysters, shucked for the asking, are consistently excellent. Eat till you're up to your ankles in 'em.

BEST FRENCH FRIES

Snuffer's (3526 Greenville, Dallas). Long, thin cuts, from fresh potatoes, with the skins still on. Crisp and brown on the outside, soft and hot on the inside. Interestingly seasoned (with garlic and onion and whatever else is in the secret formula), but just as terrific plain.

BEST FRIED ONIONS

Hog Heaven (770 Stanyan Street, San Francisco). Shredded, noncircular pieces, fried light and crisp, with love and care, from the real thing. Sweet, lacy, and full of flavor.

BEST SUZY Q'S

Sweet 16 (1534 Montana, Santa Monica). In the best drive-in tradition (Dobie Gillis never had it so good), potatoes are cut in curlicues and fried, crisp and tender, with just a smack of grease.

BEST CHEAP SEAFOOD RESTAURANT

No Name Restaurant ($15\frac{1}{2}$ Fish Pier, Boston). There's also no sign, no outside light, no decoration. Simply because there's no need. The food speaks for itself: The seafood chowder is excellent, brimming with at least a pound of fish. The clams, scallops, and salmon are as terrific as they are fresh. Even the tartar sauce—with bite-sized chunks of pickle—is homemade. Where the fishermen who catch the fish go to eat it.

BEST OFFICE BUILDING COFFEE SHOP

Mr. M's (Bender Building, 1120 Connecticut Avenue, N.W., Washington, D.C.). The secret is out: Mr. M is really Mel Krupin, owner of Mel Krupin's, a popular Washington eatery serving hard-core, uncomplicated American food. What sets this coffee shop apart is that it shares its kitchen with Krupin's more well-known restaurant, so it, too, dishes up delicious daily specials, but at a fraction of the cost. The rest of the menu—typical of the genre—isn't bad, either.

BEST PANCAKE HOUSE

Walker Bros. (153 Green Bay, Wilmette, IL; second location, Glenview). Once upon a time, a great breakfast joint became known for its pancakes, decided to remodel, brought in an extensive collection of Victorian stained glass, expanded to a second location, and through it all remembered to keep the food as good as it was at the start. Happy ending. Twenty-five years later, the show is still going strong and the cast of favorites—the chewy sourdough, the incredible oven-baked apple, and the world's best potato pancakes—still amazes. Coffee is served with pure whipping cream. No small wonder that the line often spills out the door and down the block.

BEST DRUGSTORE SODA FOUNTAIN

Highland Park Pharmacy (3229 Knox, Dallas). The shakes are just as they should be—thick, with lumps of real ice cream floating in them. The malts, freezes, floats, and phosphates are a treat, guaranteed to give your spirits a lift. The sandwiches are simple, but consistently good, with pimento cheese a specialty. There's rarely a vacant stool, but do yourself a favor and wait. This place is special, the last of a dying breed.

BEST PEANUTS

Virginia Diner (Highway 460, Wakefield, VA). Wakefield is the peanut capital of the world, and whether salted, unsalted, blanched, fresh-roasted, or raw, the nuts here are so different, so good, you won't notice that they haven't been coated in chocolate.

BEST POPCORN

Wolf's Liquor Store (1912 L Street, N.W., Washington, D.C.). Freshly popped, all day long, this is the gen-

uine stuff—like you used to get at the movies. However, capitalism sets in over the Christmas holidays, when the machine is moved out to make way for the extra booze the store hopes to sell by New Year's.

BEST BREAD PUDDING

Bon Ton Cafe (401 Magazine, New Orleans). Served warm, in a highly alcoholic whiskey sauce, with the perfect proportion of plump raisins.

BEST DEAL ON A GOURMET MEAL

Minneapolis Technical Institute (1415 Hennepin Avenue S., Minneapolis). Students training to be chefs in the commercial-foods program offer a seven-course gourmet dinner (soup to nuts) costing one-eighth of what a comparable meal would be in a downtown restaurant. An all-you-can-eat gourmet buffet is also on hand at lunch. Reservations only; dates and times vary.*

BEST RESTAURANT GIMMICK

Texas Bar-B-Que House (2401 Texas, Houston). An otherwise standard lunch of chicken or ribs is enhanced by the large wheels of fortune on both sides of this restaurant. Every day, between noon and 1:00 P.M., waitresses spin the wheels at random intervals and customers lift the vinyl tablecloths to check the right-hand table leg for a number. If the number of your table matches the number on the wheel, your lunch is free.

---

*Almost all culinary programs offer similar deals. Check your area's colleges and technical schools.

WHAT A DEAL!

ALL YOU CAN EAT

Since time began, man has searched for that perfect moment when the earth moves, firecrackers fill the sky, and at last are spoken the words he's longed to hear: "All you can eat."

Buffets and smorgasbords abound, but too often they offer either bland, predictable foods, or a high price tag where all you can eat never equals as much as you have paid for. So for something unique, incredibly priced, and best of all, where quality is valued as highly as the quantity, try . . .

The Pasta House (8213 Delmar; plus numerous other locations, St. Louis), where any day of the week the portions are gigantic (the sauces terrific) but on Monday it's also all the pasta you can eat plus bread and salad. And all you can eat is a lot, because it's not just the typical spaghetti and meatballs, but *any* pasta. You're invited—encouraged—to switch selections as often as you like on the grounds that before you go on you have to finish what you've got. For the not-so-hungry (it happens to the best of us), the restaurant will be glad to serve half-orders of any entree you request. Don't miss the toasted ravioli—a St. Louis speciality—or the pasta con broccoli, or the fettucine, or the carbonara sauce, or . . . For the Sunday bruncher, the *Manhattan Market* (1016 Second Avenue, New York) fixes a delightful one, featuring assorted smoked fish, bagels, cream cheese, herring, pastries, and wonderful, hard-crusted baguettes. But it's the last offering on the menu, "David's Cookies*— all you want," that's the clincher. . . . Tired of brunching? Head back to St. Louis, where at *The Cheshire Inn* (6306 Clayton Road) they offer a delicious alternative—an all-you-can-eat breakfast buffet (seven days a week; slightly more expensive on weekends) loaded

---

*See also WHERE TO PIG OUT: The Best of the Rest/The Cookie Hall of Fame

with hearty fare: fresh fruit, eggs, pancakes, biscuits, bacon, sausage, ham, waffles, and a few specialties such as prime-rib hash, chicken livers, and fried bananas. The only thing missing is a wheelchair to roll you out the door. . . . Once inside **R. J.'s** (252 N. Beverly Drive, Beverly Hills)—and once past the mega-dose of while-you-wait hors d'oeuvres featuring a cream cheese spread made with sour cream and chocolate chips—your attention is drawn to the spectacular "Green Grocery" salad bar, set against a backdrop of the freshest fruits and vegetables available, and lavished with over fifty items, from the basic greens, tomatoes, and cucumbers to shrimp, avocado, artichokes, and hearts of palm; an edible Garden of Eden still life that should strike joy in any pigger's heart. . . . The salad bars at **Windfield Potter's** (210 S.E. 2nd Avenue, Minneapolis) and **R. J. Grunts** (2056 Lincoln Park West, Chicago) also merit attention, as they, too, supply the pigger with enough goodies to create that rare treat—a healthy, vitamin-packed main course as rich and lush in calories as any good dessert. . . . In Baltimore, **Spittel's Half Shell** (1115 Rolling Road) offers all the crab (and beer) you can eat (and drink), until, as they say, "it backfires. . . ." **The Texas Steak Ranch and Saloon** in Houston (6009 Beverly Hill) has a "Pig-Out at the Ranch" (days and times vary, so call first) that includes soup, salad, bread, potatoes, and all the choice top sirloin you want. A meat-and-potatoes pigger's dream . . . And just for the piglets in the family, stop by California's **Griswold's Smorgasbord** (555 W. Foothill, Claremont). The bakery department has delicious home-made lollipops in such wonderful flavors as butterscotch, apple-cinnamon, and blueberry—plus enormous, flaky turnovers—but the real news is that the kids, too, get to chow down at the buffet table, where they're charged a mere thirty to thirty-five cents for each year of their age.

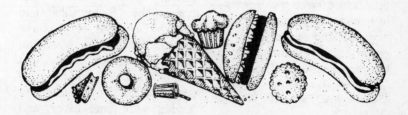

HOLY COW!

A Guide to Good, Cheap Steaks

A few choice reasons why you don't have to be as rich as Diamond Jim Brady to pig out like he did.*

THE HOFFBRAU (613 W. Sixth Street, Austin). A genuine Texas roadhouse, where the accents are for real, the decor is totally void of Southern kitsch, and the jukebox wails Willie and Waylon. Grab a table, order an ice-cold longneck, and choose from the small blackboard menu. The steaks are terrific, grilled in lemon butter, and come with German fries and a house salad of shredded lettuce mixed with olive bits in a tart, garlic-flavored dressing.

PINE CLUB (1926 Brown, Dayton, OH). No pretense here. Just a venerable steakhouse—built before the days of themes—with consistently good food. A large, rectangular bar sits in the center of the restaurant, and tables line the walls. The quality

beef, thickly cut and impeccably charred, comes with vegetables, potatoes, and a salad. The onion rings are a must. If ever a cow gave his life for a good cause, this is it.

HILLTOP STEAK HOUSE (Route US 1, Saugus, MA). This giant, raucous dinner house (it seats 1,400 at a time) with its huge neon cactus sign seems somewhat out of place in sedate New England. Lines of customers are hustled in, looking like the oversized cattle statues that dot the outside lawn. A hostess barks out table assignments, sending you to rooms with names like "Sioux City" and "Santa Fe." But once you're seated, things have a way of calming down (or maybe you just get used to it) and the pleasures begin. The steaks are tender, with great flavor, and

*See also WHO PIGS OUT: The Pigger Hall of Fame.

larger than the plates that carry them; the "dinner salad" that precedes it could feed a family of four; and rolls come with not a few pats of butter but the whole stick. Doggie bags are mandatory.

CHEROKEE SIRLOIN ROOM (886 S. Smith Street, St. Paul, MN). An informal, straightforward, friendly restaurant where no-frills comfort and terrific service are overshadowed only by an outstanding meal. The "steak of the month" is a two-inch-thick, full pound of beef, very tasty and cooked to perfection. Dinners come complete with salad, rolls, and relish dish, and the side orders really soar: the au gratin potatoes, chunky, creamy, and topped with cheddar cheese, and the onion rings, neither processed, reconstituted, nor dehydrated, but homemade and always fresh.

THE ORIGINAL PANTRY CAFE (877 S. Figueroa, Los Angeles, CA). "Never closed, never without a customer"— and never without a crowd of them waiting. But the line moves quickly, and once inside this simple Los Angeles landmark, you'll never go hungry. A bowl of iced carrots, celery, and radishes awaits you at the table. Before you can order, your waiter will appear with plates of creamy coleslaw and a huge hunk of fresh sourdough bread. These will keep you amused while you study the menu board offering gigantic portions of basic American cooking, where juicy, pan-broiled steaks and chops are the star attraction. The hash browns that accompany each order are stellar. The atmosphere is well-worn, with ceiling fans, crowded tables, and waiters who know their stuff. Huge breakfasts, too.

OH, WHAT A BEAUTIFUL MORNING

A Guide to Good, Cheap Breakfasts

In the late 1970's, during a prison riot when inmates had been holed up with their hostages for several days, the authorities finally lured them out with the smell of breakfast cooking. Breakfast was once the perfect pig-out meal for troubled economic times, essentially fresh and home-cooked, complete with generous portions and bargain prices. But the current trend toward champagne brunches has changed a lot of that, and now, finding a good, *cheap,* old-fashioned, true-blue breakfast can be maddening. Unless you know where to look.

A good place to start is at **SEARS FINE FOODS** (439 Powell Street, San Francisco), a place whose popularity is undisputed and where there isn't any choice but to order the (eighteen) miniature Swedish pancakes; the best you'll ever eat, so light they practically float off the plate, and so good you'll be tempted not to douse them in syrup. Other highlights include the strawberry waffle and the fresh fruit bowl, containing seven fruits (which vary according to the season) in an orange-juice marinade.

RAE'S (2901 Pico Blvd., Santa Monica). This turquoise diner serves a number of no-substitution combination plates; offers, in addition to the usual breakfast meats, eggs with pork chops, ham steak, and corned-beef hash; and cooks up not only one of the cheapest, but one of the best and biggest breakfasts anywhere: the "2 + 2 + 2" special, where 2 eggs, 2 pieces of bacon or sausage, 2 hot cakes or 2 biscuits—smothered in country gravy—costs just over 2 bucks.

AL'S (413 14th Avenue, S.E., Minneapolis). A cramped, narrow counter takes up nearly all of the space in what could be the world's skinniest restaurant. Drawing constant crowds from the nearby University of Minnesota, the surroundings are slightly decrepit, but the bluegrass music and terrific food—eggs, pancakes, waffles, omelets— more than compensate.

HAM AND EGGERY (530 NE 167 Street, Miami). The sign above the door reads "Welcome to Cholesterol Heaven." Bordering on shabby, this two-room, vinyl-and-plastic dive rates high for never closing, giving piggers the chance to get good breakfast grub twenty-four hours a day.

BROOKLINE LUNCH (9 Brookline Street, Cambridge, MA). Despite the name, the best meal served here is in the morn-ing. A Formica counter faces the grill, which puts out some of the best eggs around. A perfect way to add some spark to an otherwise routine day.

Author's Note: For the most cheap breakfasts per square inch, head to Las Vegas, where bacon and egg specials abound anytime, everywhere. Do avoid the 99¢-ers: It's a good bet the eggs are powdered, the fruit canned, and the potatoes frozen. For a few dollars more, any number of the big hotels—the Tropicana, the Hacienda, the Stardust—put out a memorable feast.

Five-star breakfasts—reasonably priced—are also found at both *John O'Groats* and *Lou Mitchell's* (see WHERE TO PIG OUT: The Top Ten), as well as *Duke's Coffee Shop* (see WHERE TO PIG OUT: When in Rome/A Stargazer's Guide to L.A.).

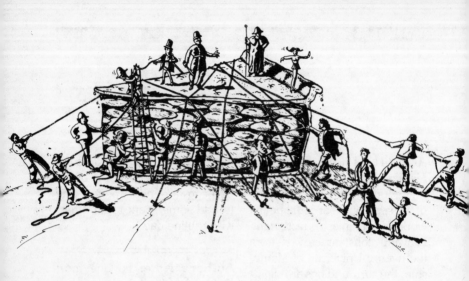

SIZE DOES MAKE A DIFFERENCE

Fed up with bite-sized portions? Then start your day at **Belisle's** (12001 Harbor Blvd., Garden Grove, CA), where the "Texas breakfast" consists of orange juice, a twenty-six-ounce top sirloin steak, twelve eggs (any style), a stack of hot cakes, country-fried potatoes, and biscuits, corn bread, or toast. . . . Still hankering for a light lunch? Head to Chicago, where at the **Bowl and Roll** (1339 N. Wells) a cup of soup is a ceramic mixing bowl with a whole boiled chicken swimming in it. . . . Need an afternoon snack, a little something to tide you over? A couple of chocolate-chip cookies from **Fuddrucker's** (3100 Chimney Rock, Houston, TX) should do the trick—they're nine inches in diameter, the size of dinner plates. . . . And speaking of dinner, you might want to go to **Fatigati's** (Old Route 50, Cuddy, PA), where they serve a hunk of prime rib with close to three pounds of meat on it. . . . Top that off with some apple pie from **More Than Just Ice Cream** (1141 Pine, Philadelphia, PA), where a single piece is actually one-fourth of the pie *or* with some chocolate cake from **R.J.'s** (252 N. Beverly Drive, Beverly Hills, CA), where each slice weighs in at a whopping three pounds. . . .

You can wash all of this down at **Lester's Diner** (State Route 84, Fort Lauderdale, FL), self-billed as the home of the fourteen-ounce cup of coffee.

LITTLE-KNOWN PIG-OUT PLACES

As advanced piggers know, pigging out is by no means restricted to "at home" or "in a restaurant." Myriad places present the pigger with opportunities for gastronomic ecstasy.

SHOPPING MALLS

There was a time when shopping malls offered weary patrons little more than family pizza parlors and ice-cream stores. But now, whole wings and floors are devoted to every kind of fast-food imaginable: At *St. Anthony Main* in Minneapolis, the **Rosebud Grocery** fills most of the bottom level with its tempting cheeses, breads, cookies, meats, salads, and desserts. At the Picnic in *Santa Monica Place* (Santa Monica, CA), stands putting out homemade potato chips (**Potatoes, Potatoes, Potatoes**), delicious, buttery grilled sandwiches (**The Incredible Toasted Sandwich**), and dozens of different gourmet cheesecakes (**Bob Busch Cheesecake**) are mixed in with the usual ethnic stalls and basic shopping-center mainstays. It's a pigger's paradise.

The obvious pinnacle of this is the likes of Boston's *Quincy Market* (at Faneuil Hall) and Baltimore's *Harborplace** (don't miss the **Boston Brownies** at either one), where huge, whole buildings have become an endless stream of restaurants, stands, stalls, vendors, and cafes, creating a glorious new world, a mini-metropolis of food. The lure of these places is that the second you have entered, you are confronted with more to eat than is possible to desire. At 10:00 A.M. or 10:00 P.M., multiple breakfast, lunch, and dinner choices abound,

---

*And more are coming: The FULTON MARKET at the South Street Seaport—in Manhattan—is currently under development, and in Kansas City, the HEARTLAND MARKET at Crown Center has just begun its first season.

although it is ridiculous even to *think* that you could digest it all in just one visit. If only, like Baskin-Robbins, they would offer little plastic spoons so you could taste. . . .

The one thing wrong with these high-tech wonders is that now the old standbys are being overlooked. A big mistake. To experience the original in heightened gluttony, drop your charge cards and spend a day (stroll, shop, munch) at the *West Side Market* (Cleveland), the *Pike Place Market* (Seattle), the *Lexington Market* (Baltimore), and the *Farmer's Market* (L.A.), where pigging out is not just fun, it's a tradition.

THE STREETS

To the pigger, the street is more than a thoroughfare for getting from one place to the next. From early May to mid-October, suburban ice-cream trucks and downtown sidewalk hot-dog carts (and all the roadside produce stands in between) spring up everywhere, transforming the local highways and byways into a makeshift open-air market. Nowhere is this more realized than in Manhattan, where along the Avenue of the Americas (Sixth Avenue), from 46th to 55th streets, a legion of street vendors offers a wonderful, cheap way to eat well. Everything you could want is found in this ten-block stretch: shish kebab, falaffel, souvlaki, tempura, and delicious cold noodles in sesame sauce (not to name them all). There's even a gourmet truck, featuring rock Cornish game hens and charcuterie from Tavern on the Green. If all this isn't enough, the show of people is unbeatable. (See also WHERE TO PIG OUT: When in Rome/A Street-Food Guide to Philadelphia.)

SPECIAL OCCASIONS

Piggers are firm believers in celebrations (they believe in anything that's an excuse to stuff their faces). Wedding receptions are a favorite—that means a lavish all-you-can-eat spread for which you won't have to pay a cent; Bar Mitzvahs follow in the tradition of the Jewish holidays—proving, once again, that less is *not* more. And *never* forget a birthday. Missing out on all that cake and ice cream would be devastating.

HAPPY HOURS

Forget the two-for-one specials and the ninety-nine-cent drinks. Serious piggers know that 4:00–7:00 P.M. at most of the better bars and lounges means a three-hour eat-a-thon of on-the-house hors d'oeuvres. Past the bowls of chips and salsa, and beyond the Swedish meatballs, there's a wide array of tasty morsels and gourmet treats just waiting to soothe your savage stomach.

Every Tuesday in St. Paul, Minnesota, at *Awada* (199 E. Plato) it's "take all you want, but eat what you take" of oysters on the half-shell and pickled herring. In Boston, *Parker's Bar* (The Parker House, 60 School Street) offers silver trays of strictly highbrow stuff: caviar, canapés, prosciutto, stuffed mushrooms, and pâté. And some of the best food in any city is at *Simply Blues* (6290 W. Sunset Blvd., Los Angeles), where you can make a meal of mini–roast-beef sandwiches and baby shrimp cocktails.

Perhaps the best things in life *are* free.

THE SUN BELT

Piggers interested in not just keeping up, but keeping ahead of the Joneses, should pack their bags and move to Phoenix, Tucson, or Corpus Christi, where new food products—such as Presto Pizza (pizza topping in a tube) and Knot-a-Bagel (bagels in the shape of a pretzel rather than a circle)—are (currently) most frequently test-marketed.

THE BEACH

Eat your heart out and get a tan while doing it. Boardwalk concessions and nearby restaurants cook up the best in fast-food fantasies: **Thrasher's** French fries (Ocean City, MD) are cut from the real thing, fried just right, and served with a heavy dose of vinegar; **Hot Dog on a Stick** at the foot of the Santa Monica Pier (Santa Monica, CA) squeezes fresh lemonade, refreshing and delicious and among the best you'll ever find; and **The White House** (Atlantic City, NJ) pleases taste buds with its superior cheesesteaks and hoagies.

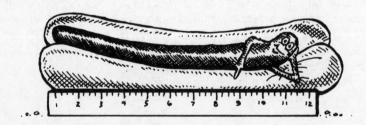

MOVIE THEATERS

The latent pigger's dream: a public place so dark that you can eat and eat and eat and no one can see what you are doing! For those of us already out of the closet, the movies offer the chance to enjoy some hard-to-find pigging favorites: bonbons, Necco wafers, Good & Plenty, and honest-to-goodness freshly popped popcorn.

STADIUMS

Some people claim to like the sport, but don't let them fool you. The real attraction here is the hot dog, plus the never-ending parade of vendors pitching peanuts, ice cream, Cracker Jack, and soda. Best of all, whatever you want can be yours without having to leave your seat.

AMUSEMENT PARKS AND CARNIVALS

Another pleasant Sunday diversion, but let's be honest: It's the cotton candy and candy apples that make it worth your while.

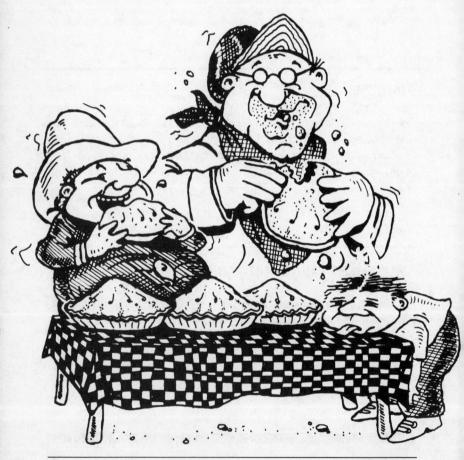

WHERE TO PIG OUT

PUT THEIR MONEY WHERE YOUR MOUTH IS
A Guide to Food-Eating Contests

What could be better than getting paid for doing what you do best?

HOT DOG–EATING CONTEST

Where:	Nathan's, Coney Island (Brooklyn, NY).
When:	Fourth of July weekend (also, Memorial Day, Labor Day).
The facts:	Winner is the contestant who consumes the most hog dogs in twelve minutes; there is a thirty-second break halfway through.
The prizes:	Certificates for free hot dogs all year long; trophies.
Contact:	Nathan's Coney Island (212) 869-0600

PUMPKIN PIE–EATING CONTEST

Where:	Pumpkin Festival (Half Moon Bay, CA).
When:	October.
The facts:	Each year, the city of Half Moon Bay holds a World Heavyweight Pumpkin Championship. Once judged, the leftover giant pumpkins are turned into pies. The winning entrant is the one who eats the most pie(s) in three minutes.
The prizes:	Ribbons.
Contact:	Terry Pimsleur & Co. 2149 Union Street San Francisco, CA 94123 (415) 346-4446

SWEET MEMORIES PIG–OUT

Where:	Sweet Memories Candy Shop (Diamond Bar, CA).
When:	Summer.
The facts:	Names of approximately fifty contestants are selected in a random drawing. For a $15.00 fee, they are given three hours to eat as much as they want of whatever they want. Whoever eats the most is declared the winner, though any sensible pigger would kill for the chance to lose.
The prizes:	A two-foot transparent glass pig filled with—what else?—candy.
Contact:	Dave Klein Sweet Memories 870 N. Diamond Bar Blvd. Diamond Bar, CA 91765 (714) 598-7242

WORLD SMELT–EATING CONTEST

Where: Kelso, WA.
When: When the smelt run (usually, the first Sunday in March).
The facts: The smelt are caught, beheaded, cleaned, and cooked. Eaters then have two hours to devour as many as they can, excluding only the bones and tail.
The prizes: Steak dinners, large trophies.
Contact: Kelso Eagle Lodge
530 27th Street
Kelso, WA 98626
(206) 425-8330

OYSTER–EATING CONTEST

Where: Milford, CT.
When: Sunday of the third weekend in August.
The facts: A National Oyster Shucking Contest is held every year in Milford. Once all the oysters have been so perfectly opened, *somebody* has to eat them. The winner is the fastest eater of thirty oysters.
The prizes: $25.00/$10.00.
Contact: Chamber of Commerce
P.O. Box 452
Milford, CT 06460
(203) 878-0681

FROG–EATING CONTEST

Where: Rayne, LA.
When: September.
The facts: Definitely a gourmet event: The affair begins with numerous bottles of wine and toasts; the table is set with fresh flowers and the finest china, silver, linen, and crystal. Each entrant is given fifteen minutes to eat as many frog legs as possible, though judging is based not only on the quantity he consumes but on the elegance of his manners as well. Rules also stipulate that each time a frog leg is eaten, the contestant must announce the fact by uttering an audible "ribbit."
The prizes: An engraved plaque (proclaiming "King Frog Eater").
Contact: Chamber of Commerce
P.O. Box 383
Rayne, LA 70578
(318) 334-2332
[By invitation only . . .]

After she lost an eating contest to five-foot one-inch, 422-pound Dee Dee Spencer, five-foot two-inch, 375-pound Emma "Big Bertha" Creighton commented, "I made a big mistake. I turned to the tapioca pudding after the hot food, and Dee Dee went after the tuna salad. Tapioca pudding—which is one of my favorites—is no match in calories for tuna salad, with all that mayo in it." The twenty-eight-year-old winner consumed 42,194 calories in a five-hour period—eating more than the average person consumes in two and one-half weeks.

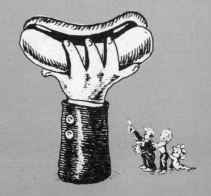

TRADE SECRETS

A Guide to Guided Tours

Attention Piggers: Recent studies have shown that people who eat chocolate are less likely to suffer from tooth decay because the cocoa butter in chocolate coats their teeth, forming a protective seal.

To learn more about your loved ones—and for the chance to walk away with your pockets stuffed with them—here's a list of companies who will show you how they do it.

SARA LEE, 500 Waukegan Road, Deerfield, IL; (312) 945-2525. Free tour available 10:00 A.M.–1:00 P.M., Monday–Friday. Lasts one and a half hours. Reservations necessary. Highlight is the Hospitality Room, where guests are taken at the end of the tour to taste the cakes and Danish.

HERSHEY CHOCOLATE COMPANY, Hershey, PA; (717) 534-4900. For safety and quality-assurance reasons, Hershey's discontinued their tour of the plant in 1973. They have set up a free visitor center (open 9:00 A.M.–4:45 P.M., Monday–Saturday) which includes an automated ride through displays

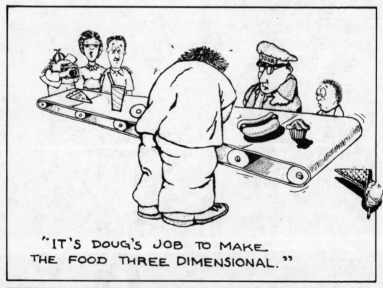

"IT'S DOUG'S JOB TO MAKE THE FOOD THREE DIMENSIONAL."

depicting the story of chocolate, as well as an historical exhibit, dessert cafe, souvenir shop, and candy counter. No free samples. However, the Hershey plant in Oakdale, CA (an hour east of San Francisco) *does* let you inside the plant, from 8:15 A.M.–3:30 P.M., Monday–Friday. The free tour is one-half hour in length and, in the tradition of the old Pennsylvania factory tour, comes complete with free candy samples. Call (209) 847-0381.

NABISCO, Fair Lawn Bakery, 211 Route 208, Fairlawn, NJ; (201) 797-6800. Free tours available from October through May. Includes trip through mixing and baking areas, where you watch the product go in and out, then pass through quality control and into packaging. Guests leave with a complimentary package of cookies or crackers.

BETTY CROCKER, P.O. Box 1113, Minneapolis, MN; (612) 540-2526. Free tours available 10:00 A.M.–3:00 P.M., Monday–Friday. Begins every hour on the hour. Guests are taken through the seven test kitchens, where they might witness tolerance tests or preparation of food for promotional, cookbook, and package photographs. Morning tours are preceded by coffee and sweet rolls, while coffee and cookies

are served to afternoon guests. Each guest is also presented with a free gift package when he leaves. Reservations requested.

STANDARD CANDY COMPANY, P.O. Box 101025, Nashville, TN. Two free tours available daily; write ahead for times and scheduling. A chance to see how Goo Goo Clusters are made. Freebies, too.

PEPPERIDGE FARM, bakery at 595 Westport Avenue, Norwalk, CT; (203) 846-7246. Free tour given 12:00–4:00 P.M., Sunday only. Lasts one-half hour. See the bakery in action and walk away with samples.

KRÖN CHOCOLATIER, 37 E. 18 Street, New York; (212) 982-4850. "A chocolate workshop," by appointment only. For $25.00, guests are taken on a tour of the factory by Thomas Krön, the company's founder. Included is a lecture on the history of chocolate and chocolate making and the chance to watch the process from start to finish. Guests are encouraged to use their fingers—sampling is permitted—and are given the opportunity to both taste off the conveyor belt and mold their own chocolate. A special "goody bag" is presented to each visitor before leaving.

AROUND THE WORLD IN LESS THAN A DAY

A Guide to Special Events Highlighting Ethnic Foods

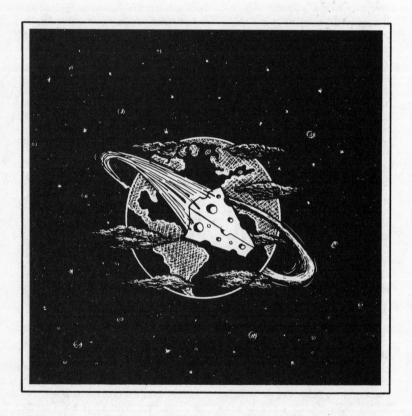

A TASTE OF CHICAGO runs for a four-day period over the Fourth of July holiday. Seventy-five different Chicago-area restaurants dish up their specialties at a picnic in Grant Park. Admission is free, and food prices range from 50¢ to $3.00. Music to suit everyone's taste and a spectacular fireworks show as well. A "mini-taste" is now being held over Labor Day weekend. (312) 644-7430.

LOS ANGELES STREET SCENE, held the second weekend in October in the downtown area surrounding City Hall, features over 100 vendors and concessions offering a wide variety of ethnic foods, representative of all nationalities and races. No admission charge. (213) 485-5801.

NINTH AVENUE INTERNATIONAL FOOD FESTIVAL, in New York City, runs a mile along Ninth Avenue from 37th to 57th streets. Held in May, the weekend following Mother's Day, it involves the area's merchants, community groups, and residents, as well as outside vendors, who offer food, from over forty nations. Arts and crafts are also available. (212) 581-7029.

FEAST OF SAN GENNARO is New York City's oldest festival, a ten-day eating extravaganza held on Mulberry Street from Park Street to E. Houston. It usually starts between the second and third week of November, but exact date does vary. This is a charitable (not commercial) venture, and while some ethnic dishes are available, it is mostly Italian cooking, with over 200 vendors on hand. Mamma mia! (212) 226-9546.

HOLIDAY FOLK FAIR, sponsored by the International Institute in Milwaukee, is without a doubt *the* great ethnic pig-out. The fun takes place the Friday, Saturday, and Sunday before Thanksgiving, at the MECCA Convention Hall. Includes folk dancing, cultural exhibits, and crafts, but the International Sidewalk Cafe—featuring over 300 different foods—is alone worth the price of admission. (414) 933-0521.

PITTSBURGH FOLK FESTIVAL is sponsored by Robert Morris College and held the Friday, Saturday, and Sunday of Memorial Day weekend. This ethnic fair showcases thirty different nationalities through dance and homemade foods. It takes place on Fifth Avenue at Sixth, and there is a small admission charge. (412) 227-6812.

WHAT YOU SEE
IS WHAT YOU GET

Make no mistake about what these places serve to eat.

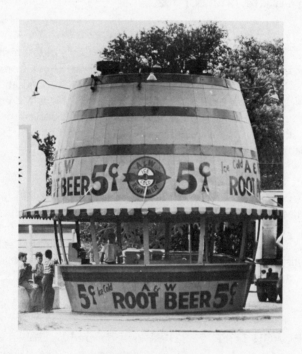

A & W
(location unknown)
Fresno, California

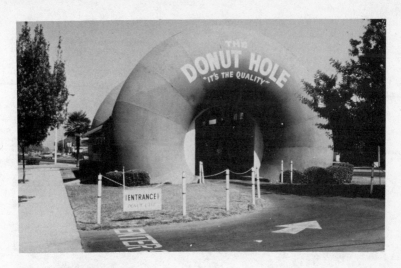

THE DONUT HOLE
15300 E. Amar Road
La Puente, California

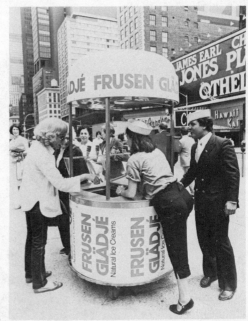

FRUSEN GLÄDJÉ
ICE CREAM
Street cart
New York, New York

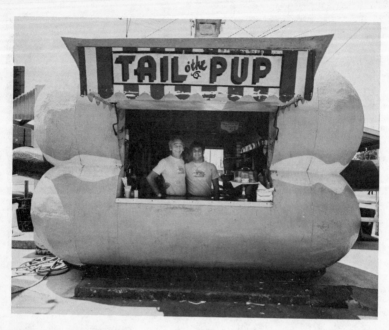

TAIL O' THE PUP
311 N. La Cienega Boulevard
Los Angeles, California

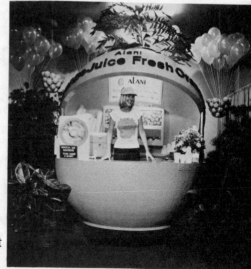

ALANI
Lobby,
Moisant International Airport
New Orleans, Louisiana

WHEN IN ROME

How to Do Like the Locals Do

A BARBECUE GUIDE TO TEXAS

There's good barbecue all over Texas, from corner stands to fancy places. And while it's somewhat difficult to mess up good beef just by smoking it, there are those that clearly rise above the rest.

In *Houston,* a good choice is **GOODE COMPANY** (5109 Kirby), a one-of-a-kind Texas bunkhouse filled with tractor seats and beer signs, and with antlers doubling as handles on the screen doors. The meat is moist and tender and the sauce is on the sweet side, the latter a sure sign that you are, indeed, in east Texas. . . . A real hole-in-the-wall place, with vinyl chairs, Formica tables, and a well-worn linoleum floor, is the **SHEPHERD DRIVE BARBECUE** stand (1703 N. Shepherd), where the sliced-beef sandwich is loaded with wonderfully crusty edges and served on the only kind of bread on which to eat a barbecue sandwich—the kind that sticks to the roof of your mouth. . . . If you prefer a sauce without the thick sweetness of a tomato base, try the **LULING CITY MARKET** (4726 Richmond), where central-Texas barbecue has finally come to Houston. Pseudo-western decor aside, you order meat-market style—buy as little or as much as you want, and pay not by the plate but by the pound, receiving the whole mess wrapped up in a sheet of reddish-brown butcher paper. The pork ribs are quite good, and while the beef sometimes has a tendency to dry out, the crust is exceptional.

Piggers in *Dallas* should count their blessings. The barbecue at both **SONNY BRYAN'S** and **ANGELO'S** is so good, you'll swear it has healing powers. (See WHERE TO PIG OUT: The Top Ten.)

A TEX–MEX GUIDE TO TEXAS

Ninfa's, 2704 Navigation, Houston; plus other locations. What began as a hole-in-the-wall, ten-table barrio restaurant in 1973 (converted from a failing tortilla factory) has branched into a restaurant chain which is now as fashionable to put down as it once was to praise. Still, certain items—the queso appetizer, the green table salsa, the tacos à la Ninfa (soft tacos filled with strips of char-broiled skirt steak)—are as good as they were at the start; the very foundation Tex-Mex was built on.

Dallas Tortilla & Tamale Factory, 2717 N. Harwood, Dallas. Tucked away on a side street in a part-industrial, part-residential area, this place is indeed what the name promises . . . a factory. There are no seats, and food is sold by the bulk—"to go," over the counter only—with prices so low that even when you can't possibly eat it all, it's impossible not to order anyway. Tamales, in six different variations, are boxed in groups of twelve; each day, there are fresh jalapeño, chorizo, Mexican sauce, and cheese. On weekends, the crowds line up for the homemade barbecoa (Mexican barbecue—a calf's head, wrapped in a sack, and cooked in a pit until tender) and the gallon jugs of menudo (a Mexican beef soup made with tripe and hominy).

But the best menudo, aficionados will tell you, is at *Los Arcos Cafe,* 502 S. Zarzamora, San Antonio, where this specialty of the house is so well known it isn't even listed on the menu.

Also in San Antonio, don't miss *Mi Tierra Cafe and Bakery,* 218 Produce Row, El Mercado. A landmark, this twenty-four-hour operation offers the best selection of Mexican breads, pastries, and candy as well as a host of other foods. And if tacos are your thing, *Texas Hot Stuff,* 2915 Frio City Road, has dozens to consider (the tortillas are made fresh in the restaurant), ranging from bacon and egg to barbecoa to carne guisada (a stewed beef).

Visit **Su Casa,** 6901 Capitol, Houston, for the best stock of Mexican beers, not to mention terrific tacos al carbón; all in a perfectly ramshackle ambience, thankfully lacking in pretense and light on the theme decor.

In Dallas, **Guadalajara,** 3308 Ross, has much the same feel; the entrees—enchiladas, tamales, chiles rellenos—are basic, but dependably good; the sopapillas, dripping in honey, are a joy. Particularly at 3:00 in the morning.

Open twenty-four hours, the best time to pig out at **Las Cazuelas,** 2219 Fulton, Houston, is also after midnight, on the weekends, when the crowd is at its liveliest. This is an authentic Mexican taqueria, complete with glassed-in kitchen (so you can see the food as it's prepared), crazed mariachis, an un-Americanized menu, and racks of Spanish magazines, records, and tapes. All very much like you've left the country and gone south . . . *way* south.

In Texas, tracking down a good "bowl of red" is not as easy as you'd expect, a funny thing in a state under constant threat of fire from all the chili being cooked off. **Tolbert's** (4544 McKinney, Dallas) and **Crazy Ed's** (13855 Highway 59, Sugar Land) are both operated by past winners of state chili championships and both serve up a blend that's meaty, robust, and full-flavored. . . . But, despite its chain status, the best of the best is at **Chili's** (locations statewide): sinus-clearing, blood-pumping, and so fiery that it will bring tears of joy to your eyes.

(For die-hard chili-heads, the *Goat Gap Gazette* lets loose on everything you wanted to know about a bowl of red but were afraid to ask, including up-to-the-minute information on cookoffs, winners, and related events. Contact 5110 Bayard Lane, #2, Houston, TX 77006 for subscription details.)

A "DELI" GUIDE TO NEW YORK

Best Pastrami and Corned Beef: **Carnegie Delicatessen** (854 Seventh Avenue at 55th). One of the few places that still bothers to make their own, and it shows ... Best Chopped Liver: **Wolf's Delicatessen** (corner Avenue of the Americas and 57th). Moist, with the right hit of chicken fat. Better than what mother used to make, this is like *grandmother* used to make ... Best Knishes: **Yonah Schimmel** (137 E. Houston). Tasty and remarkably unleaden ... Best Bagels: **H & H Bagels** (2239 Broadway at 80th); **Jumbo Hot Bagels** (1068 Second Avenue). Where the restaurants and bakeries get theirs. Hot and fresh, and open twenty-four hours a day ... Best Rye Bread: **The Cellar** at Macy's (135 W. 34th Street); **Zabar's** (249 W. 80th Street). With caraway seeds, with black seeds, and with a wonderfully chewy crust ... Best Cheesecake*: **Junior's Delicatessen** (386 Flatbush Avenue, Brooklyn). Smooth and rich and unsurpassed. Certainly worth the hassle of getting to Brooklyn, but what a lot of piggers don't know is that it's also available at Barton's candy stores throughout Manhattan, as well as through the mail. (See also HOW TO PIG OUT: How to Pig Out When There's Nothing in the House/Mail-Order Pig-Out.) ... Best Dairy Restaurant: **B & H Dairy Luncheonette** (127 Second Avenue). A dinky, cramped counter, a couple of tables; excellent blintzes, potato soup, and challah French toast, the latter so generously smothered with butter and egg it will drive a cholesterol level into ecstasy ... Best All-Around Deli: **2nd Avenue Delicatessen** (156 Second Avenue at 10th). For atmosphere, price, and food. If the sandwiches were stacked any higher they would be hazardous to air-traffic control. Great soups, too.

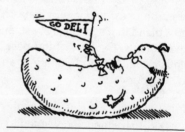

*Gourmet cheesecakes—marble, white chocolate, and flavored with liqueurs—also abound in New York. The best of these is at **Miss Grimble's** (305 Columbus Avenue), a bakery (not a deli), but pigging heaven all the same.

A GUIDE TO
OLD NEW YORK

East Side,
West Side . . .
a look at some
pigging classics.

Horn & Hardart Automat (200 E. 42nd Street). Sure, it's bland cafeteria food, but this fabled dining institution is the last of its kind. And who can resist the little doors and the art-deco vending machines? Besides, they now sell David's Cookies.

Katz's Delicatessen (205 E. Houston). The epitome of deli atmosphere; huge, lively, and inexpensive. Enormous sandwiches, the world's best hot dogs (see WHERE TO PIG OUT: Best Bets/Top Dog[s]).

Ray's Pizza (465 Avenue of the Americas). The first New York pizzeria opened at $53\frac{1}{2}$ Spring Street in 1895, and today there is certainly no dearth of good pizza in Manhattan. It is everywhere, whole or—a New York specialty—by the slice. And the best slice is at Ray's: slightly oily, with wonderfully stringy cheese, good sauce, and a crust that's crisp and chewy.

Dave's Luncheonette (416 Broadway). You can order a sandwich or hot dog if you like, but the star attraction here is the egg cream—the *real* thing, down to the homemade syrup. The very stuff pigging legends were made of.

Dubrow's Cafeteria (515 Seventh Avenue). See WHERE TO PIG OUT: Best Bets/Self-Serve.

Supreme Macaroni (511 Ninth Avenue). This typically dark and dusty storefront, lined with wooden bins filled with macaroni and noodles, holds an unexpected surprise in the back. A small, cheerful Italian restaurant with good food and reasonable prices. A real find.

WHERE

THE STARS PIG

A Stargazer's Guide to L.A.

Duke's Coffee Shop (at the Tropicana Motel, 8585 Santa Monica Blvd.). "Your mother wants you to eat your breakfast" is emblazed across the menu. And with good reason. There are egg dishes and three-egg omelets too numerous to count; the best blintzes in town; hot cakes with apples, blueberries, or bananas; an extravagant mix of fresh fruit served in a bowl; and toast that's "burnt on request." All of this in a dive of a coffee shop, with a counter and long tables laid end to end, which you usually end up sharing with strangers. No matter; the clientele is an amusing mix, and even if you don't recognize a familiar face amid the musicians, actors, agents, writers, and studio executives, the small freezer by the cash register houses frozen Milky Ways and Hershey bars that will surely make you leave with a smile. As will the huge portions and low prices. Great club sandwiches, too.

Lucy's Cafe El Adobe (5536 Melrose Avenue). You'll know this one by the larger-than-life-sized picture of Jerry Brown in the window. The basic two-room restaurant is a local political pit stop and in a prime location—directly across the street from Paramount Studios. The food doesn't hurt, either; consistently good items include the arroz con pollo, the barbecued-beef taco and tostada, and the margaritas—frothy, without the slush, and quietly stiff. All in all, pleasant, relaxing, and welcomingly understated.

Schwab's (8024 W. Sunset Blvd.). Whether Lana Turner was discovered here or not really doesn't matter; this combination drugstore/coffee shop/soda fountain is an on-target blend of tradition, tackiness, and importance. The waitresses are pleasantly abrupt, treating everyone equally, whether famous or unknown. Nowhere else can you hole up in a gold vinyl booth to order a peanut-butter and jelly sandwich and a chocolate shake. Good eggs and onions, too.

Colony Coffee Shop (23706 W. Pacific Coast Highway, Malibu). This is Schwab's gone west, a bare-bones coffee shop housed in the Malibu Pharmacy, where the local elite gather to meet and eat. So, no need to plot your way past the Colony guard anymore. Just grab a seat and order some breakfast or a burger, knowing that even if you can't afford to live next door to a star,

sooner or later you'll be pigging out with one.

Piggers who strike out at all of the above need not head for the nearest map seller or book a tour by bus. The best of the local delis—*Art's* (12224 Ventura Blvd., Studio City), *Greenblatt's* (8017 Sunset Blvd.), *Nate 'n Al's* (414 N. Beverly Drive, Beverly Hills), and *Canter's* (419 N. Fairfax Blvd.) are all potential sighting sites. Just remember to keep your eyes open between bites.

A GUIDE TO DOWN–HOME COOKING

MARY MAC'S, 228 Ponce De Leon, N.E., Atlanta. A rambling restaurant, combining the best of Southern hospitality with Yankee efficiency. The decor is basic: You are seated at a Formica-topped table in one of four dining rooms and asked to write your own order. Dinner translates to one "meat," and four choices from among the vegetables, salads, and desserts. Selections change daily, but include such regional favorites as chicken-pan pie, country-fried steak,

black-eyed peas, and pot likker (the liquid left in the bottom of the greens pot, which is poured into a bowl, topped with crumbled corn bread, and eaten like soup). This is food like old Aunt Bessie used to cook . . . assuming, of course, that Aunt Bessie was a very good cook.

LEISURE BOARDING HOUSE & DINER, 219 S. Randall, Pasadena, TX. You're not going to believe this one. A genuine boardinghouse, serving food so good that they've had to expand the dining room several times in order to handle the crowds. Piggers sit elbow-to-elbow at long tables; platters piled high with chicken, meat loaf, mashed potatoes, veggies, and hot rolls are passed around family-style. Everyone pays the same price, regardless of what you want or how much you eat. The atmosphere is friendly, but strictly business; a sign on the cash register reads "Yes, we take no checks and the bank don't fry no chicken." Wonderful breakfasts, too, from 5:30 A.M. to 9:00 A.M.

DEACON BURTON'S SOUL FOOD CAFE, Edgewood and Hurt, S.E., Atlanta. It's doubtful that you could eat any better than this at home, and you certainly couldn't eat any cheaper. Service is cafeteria-style, from 4:00 A.M. to 4:00 P.M. (except Sunday), and the meals are hearty and filling. Other than an occasional pig's ear, however, the accent is more country than soul, with excellent meat loaf, chicken and dumplings, biscuits, and greens. You pay by the plate, extra if you want dessert (usually pound cake or fresh cobbler). Trust me, you want dessert.

THE BISHOP GRILL, 308 N. Bishop, Dallas. An unprepos-

sessing lunchroom, off the beaten path, in the Oak Cliff section of town. Food is dished out in makeshift cafeteria-fashion; for a set price, you choose a main course, such as smothered steak or chicken, and anywhere from one to three side dishes (okra, zucchini, peas, macaroni . . .) to go with it. The outstanding homemade rolls disprove the old adage "Don't fill up on bread"; they're so incredible that you'd be a fool not to. (A mile or two away a second place, **ROSE-MARIE'S,** 1411 N. Zangs, offers the same food from the same kitchen but in roomier surroundings.)

AUNT FANNY'S CABIN, 375 Campbell Road, Smyrna, GA. Outside Atlanta, this is authentic Southern cooking, complete with the authentic Southern-dinner treatment. Black children recite the menu, and huge women dressed in plantation regalia serve family-style dinners. There's a touch of gimmick, but it's sincere, and the fried chicken and Smithfield ham are among the best there is. Bowls of fresh vegetables and baskets of biscuits will keep you happy. The corn bread will drive you out of your mind.

DURGIN-PARK, 340 Faneuil Hall Marketplace, Boston. "Established before you were born," and little has changed on the menu in the last 135 years. Ascend the stairs to the dining rooms one flight up, with their long communal tables, red-and-white-checkered cloths, mustard-colored walls, and waitresses who won't hesitate to tell you what they think. The food is abundant and robust; truly Yankee cooking at its best. Big, thick slabs of rare roast beef, beans, chowder, Indian pudding, and an apple pan dowdy any pigger would kill for. No reservations and always a line. Always worth waiting for, too.

LOUISE'S PANTRY, 124 South Palm Canyon Drive, Palm Springs, CA. Any hour of the day, any day of the week, the front stoop of this vintage 1940's bungalow is overflowing with people—locals and tourists—eagerly awaiting their turn to chow down on some terrific home-style food. The menu features a full offering of basic American cooking, but while the burgers and club sandwiches take a backseat to the delicious daily specials (ample five-course meals featuring pork chops, chicken and dumplings, roast beef and gravy), the best has appropriately been saved for last. Don't overlook the homemade cakes and pies (two points for the

chocolate cream), pigging proof that there's more to Palm Springs than polyester pants and charity tennis tournaments. (Closed during summer, June 15–September 15.)

A STREET-FOOD GUIDE TO PHILADELPHIA

Cheesesteaks. The pillar of Philadelphia fast-foods. **JIM'S STEAKS** is the stand-out (see WHERE TO PIG OUT: Best Bets/The Sandwich Hall of Fame), but **PAT'S, KING OF STEAKS** (1237 E. Passayunk) is also good, not only for local color and a great sandwich, but for a bit of movie history: "Rocky" ate here. Trapped in the Jersey suburbs? Not as hopeless as you might think. **BIG JOHN'S** (1800 E. Marlton Pk., Cherry Hill, NJ) fixes up a cheesesteak so deliciously sloppy you'll swear you never left Center City.

Italian Water Ices. This combination of shaved ice and fruit syrups is generally available only in the summer, when it is sold by concessions everywhere. The top of the line comes from **OVERBROOK** (stands at 5901 Turner; 4369 Main), where the lemon, in particular, tastes more like lemons than . . . lemons.

Soft Pretzels.* Hot, doughy, salty, and best with mustard. Available from vendors throughout the city, but if you want them fresh from the oven, go straight to the source: **THE FEDERAL PRETZEL CO.** (638 Federal), or **PHILADELPHIA SOFT PRETZEL** (4315 3rd Street). Get there early; these factories sell out fast.

Hoagies. The lifeblood of the hoagie is the sauce, serving as a bridge between the bread and the meat, and giving an otherwise standard submarine sandwich its distinctive favor and character. The king of sauces— and hence the best hoagie—is at **LEE'S** (44 S. 17th Street; plus other locations), where the ingredients are one of Philadelphia's best-kept secrets. Nevertheless, whatever is in it, it will keep you coming back for more.

---

*According to legend, the distinctive twist of the pretzel is said to be representative of a child's arms folded in prayer; probably because in seventh-century France, monks in the monastery gave pretzels to schoolchildren as a reward for learning their religious lessons. Oddly enough, all pretzels were originally soft. Hard pretzels didn't come about until later—and by accident—when a baker fell asleep and the batch he was preparing was left for too long in the oven.

AN ORIENTAL-FOOD GUIDE TO SAN FRANCISCO

In San Francisco, choosing an Oriental restaurant can be a problem. They all have Formica-topped tables, too-bright fluorescent lighting, and off-white dinnerware with a nondescript pattern running around the rim. At the more elaborate places, the food may be terrific, but the cost of pigging out is doubled because somebody has to pay for the interior decorator. And dare you just walk off the street into any restaurant at random, you will most likely end up with a boring plate of Cantonese food and an overdose of MSG.

Not to worry. More and more, there is great Oriental pigging going on in the Avenues, an area on the west side of the city (north of Golden Gate Park) that is beginning to out-Chinatown Chinatown. Obviously, you should hit at least one neighborhood or the other, though any pigger knows that the best rule is the oldest: One from Column A, one from Column B. Hence:

Column A (Chinatown)

YUET LEE
1300 Stockton Street
Best: all seafood dishes.

YA SU YUAN
638 Pacific Street
Best: Manchurian beef, prawns in egg-white sauce.

MANDARIN DELIGHT
941 Kearny Street
Best: any diced pork dish. (Try the "ants on a tree.")

CHUCK'S FOUNTAIN
999 Powell Street
A funky neighborhood hangout, complete with soda fountain.
Best: the Chinese beef stew with homemade wonton and boiled noodles.

ASIA GARDEN
772 Pacific Street*
Clearly the place to see and be seen in Chinatown.
Best: Dim Sum.

Column B (the Avenues)

OCEAN
726 Clement Street
Lines so long, they've had to open a second place a few blocks down; menu sounds uninspired, but food merits the crowds.
Best: everything.

TSING TAO
3107 Clement Street
Best: anything (including wonderful fried dishes).

GOLDEN TURTLE
308 5th Avenue (Vietnamese)
Best: beef, shrimp, or chicken made with lemongrass.

KHAN TOKE THAI HOUSE
5937 Geary Blvd.
Quite simply, Thai food at its best.

*Don't even *think* of missing this one.

A DEEP-DISH PIZZA GUIDE TO CHICAGO

Ike Sewell opened **Pizzeria Uno** (29 E. Ohio)* in 1943, creating a Chicago legend—the thick-crusted, deep-dish pizza. And though in recent years his operation has been busy going national, the quality here remains true to the original—genuine knife-and-fork pizza, with imported mozzarella and Parmesan, lots of fresh sausage, and a sauce made with tomatoes and not merely tomato sauce. . . . At **Gino's East** (160 E. Superior), the sign says "World's Finest Pizza," and indeed, the special cornmeal crust—light and crunchy, less yeasty and heavy—is perfection. . . . One of the best pizzas outside the city is at **Nancy's** (940 N. York, Elmhurst), where urbanites will find the Sicilian spinach pie, with its double crust and chunky, creamy spinach-and-cheese filling, worth a drive to the suburbs. . . . For piggers seeking something different, **The Chicago Pizza and Oven Grinder** (2121 N. Clark) offers a new twist: sauce, mushrooms, and assorted ingredients are combined in a bowl, covered with a thick crust, and then baked, creating a sort of upside-down, inside-out pizza. . . . But the most inventive deep-dish trend is the stuffed ("twin") pizza at **Giordano's** (747 N. Rush; plus other locations). It starts out simple enough—a combination of dough, fresh mushrooms, spicy sausage, and mozzarella—but then a second crust is added and that, in turn, is topped with a mild tomato sauce and a layer of Parmesan and Romano cheeses; all in all, a noted pigging achievement. . . . **Bacino's** (2204 N. Lincoln) also serves a stuffed pizza, and here's where the story gets interesting. There used to be a Giordano's where Bacino's is now, and the pizza is remarkably similar. But if Bacino's is a Giordano's clone, it's done them one better—better sauce, fresher ingredients, a less doughy crust, plus the identical-sized pizza is less expensive; bite for bite, dollar for dollar, the number one in town.

---

*A second restaurant, **Pizzeria Due** (619 N. Wabash), followed later.

A GUIDE TO SOME SPECIAL SPECIALTIES

In *Buffalo,* chicken wings are an institution, served in every bar, tavern, pub, restaurant, and pizza parlor. But nobody makes them better than the **ANCHOR BAR** (1047 Main Street). Halved wings, looking like tiny drumsticks, are deep-fried, then coated with a buttery, hot sauce, and served with celery sticks and a special blue-cheese dressing. The combination of foods—the crispness and juice of the chicken, the fire of the sauce, and the cool of the celery and dressing—is a delicious ménage à trois of flavors.

In *Cincinnati,* **SKYLINE CHILI** (643 Vine Street; numerous other locations) dishes out Cincinnati chili, which has nothing to do with Texas chili, but is a pigging pleasure all its own. It comes plain, or in combinations—"2-way," "3-way," "4-way," or "5-way," the last of which is a bowl of spaghetti, topped with chili, beans, chopped onions, and grated cheese.

In *Kansas City,* no trip is complete without a stop at **AR-THUR BRYANT'S BARBE-CUE** (1727 Brooklyn), where the ribs and fries are legendary, but it's the sauce that put Kansas City on the international pigging map. Ten-gallon jugs filled with the stuff bathe in the filtered sunlight breaking through the dusty front window. Reddish-orange in color, it is rich, thick, and tangy, leaning toward hot, and without a ketchupy taste. The spices are a wonderful blend of everything from curry to cayenne. (In December 1982, Arthur Bryant died of a heart attack at age 80. Essentially a one-man operation, Bryant's "House of Good Eats" is now being run by his daughter. We can only hope that the famous sauce will live on.)

THE TOP TEN

You can please some of the piggers all of the time and all of the piggers some of the time; however, at each of the following, all of the piggers are pleased all of the time. The Loving Spoonful Awards go to:

THE APPLE PAN
10801 W. Pico Blvd.
Los Angeles, CA

This white wooden diner, with its U-shaped counter, ceiling fans, paneled walls, and freshly baked pies lining the kitchen window, has been serving the definitive in pig-out foods since 1947. And not a one of them disappoints. The burgers are legendary, messy, and full of flavor, slathered with mayonnaise, pickles, lettuce, cheese, and a "special" sauce deserving that word; the tuna, egg salad, and ham sandwiches are equally as good—and unequaled anywhere else; and the pies—apple, banana, pecan, pumpkin, and boysenberry cream, among others—are a tribute to great American cooking (one bite and you're guaranteed to hear bells). But not only is it what is served here, it's the way that it's served: by frenetic countermen in long aprons and soda-jerk hats, doing six things at once and never missing a beat; and on old-fashioned diner china, with water in pointed paper cups (that wilt by the time you're ready to leave)

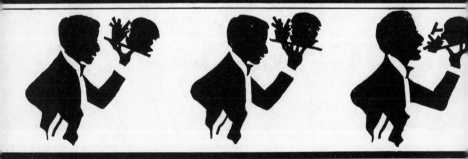

and soft drinks not by the glass but by the bottle. The sign outside says "Quality Forever." They aren't kidding.

THE CAMELLIA GRILL
626 S. Carrollton
New Orleans, LA

A taste of tradition with a dollop of Southern charm. You'll feel like Blanche DuBois as you sweep your way past the grand white columns and the mini-plantation exterior. Inside, a maître d' greets you and shows you to your seat—one of twenty-nine stools at a counter. Waiters dutifully dish out any number of excellent breakfasts, blue-plate specials, sandwiches, and burgers, all while incongruously dressed in formal dinner jackets and black bow ties.

What's more, even the napkins are linen—all the better, you'll discover, for wiping your mouth after chowing down on a Cannibal Special (a one-of-a-kind steak tartare sandwich made with raw ground meat, onion, and egg and served on a terrific rye) and a hunk of pecan pie. (See also WHERE TO PIG: The Best of the Rest/Best Pie.) Located at the end of the streetcar line, this popular little eatery is everything any pigger could desire.

CYRANO'S
1059 S. Big Bend
St. Louis, MO

Tuxedoed waiters, fresh flowers, marble-topped tables, classical music. The red-carpet treatment, all right, but looks can be deceiv-

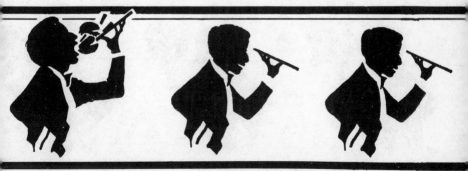

ing. Not a single pea-sized, over-priced, overrated nouvelle-cuisine dish in sight. This is hard-core stuff. For starters, try the onion soup (with a wonderfully crusty layer of Gruyère cheese) or the Cyrano's Special, thick slices of rare roast beef on a hard French roll, the top of the nondeli line. Both are excellent, but eating dinner here would still be an experience if only as an excuse to work your way to (and through) what could be the best dessert selection in the country. The Cleopatra, as enticing as its namesake, is irresistible, a statuesque serving of French vanilla ice cream in a rich chocolate shell that has been surrounded by sliced bananas and halved fresh strawberries and topped with a mound of whipped cream. The World's Fair Éclair, the bananas flambé, the caramel custard, the *gâteau cho-* *colat,* the Black Forest cake (*especially* the Black Forest cake), the baba au rhum—each is a work of art, an alluring combination of elegance and beauty, gluttony and greed. And wait, there's more: Not only are the portions staggering and the prices affordable, but amid all this opulence they don't expect you to sacrifice pigging comfort; there are no silly pretensions about having to dress up for the food. Truly the best of both worlds: pigging with a touch of class.

JOHN O'GROATS
BREAKFAST AND LUNCH
10516 W. Pico Blvd.
Los Angeles, CA

The only thing wrong with this homey counter-style restaurant is that it isn't open for dinner. Ev-

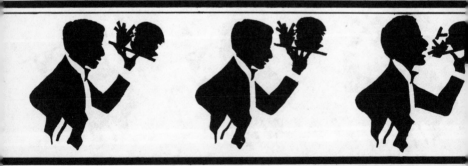

erything is fresh and lovingly cooked to order, and it shows—from the baking-powder biscuits, the perfectly turned eggs, and the French toast flavored with cinnamon and vanilla, to the mouthwatering shortbread and the amazingly crisp, amazingly greaseless (amazingly low-priced) fried chicken and fish and chips. Housed in a grey stucco cottage with blue and white wallpaper and lace curtains, the feel here is warm and comfortable, more like an overgrown country kitchen than a restaurant. When can you remember a restaurant making hot chocolate with real milk or, better yet, pouring refills straight from the saucepan in which it was made? The guy in the kitchen is owner Bob Jacoby; his wife, Angie, is the heart-of-gold waitress behind the counter. Their place is a gem.

JOHN'S PIZZERIA
278 Bleecker
New York, NY

If pizza is a New York institution, then this cramped Greenwich Village establishment, which dishes out whole pies only, should be declared a landmark. The combination of dough, cheese, sauce, spices (get garlic), and toppings is unequaled, a perfect blend of flavors where nothing overpowers. And cooked the way it should be, in a stone-floor, coal-burning oven, so that the crust comes out blistered and charred around the edges. The decor, too, is what you would expect—basic pizzeria, with bare booths, wooden tables, paper napkins, and canned soda. There's good reason that even in bad weather or despite the long lines, people are willing to wait: Plain and simple, this is

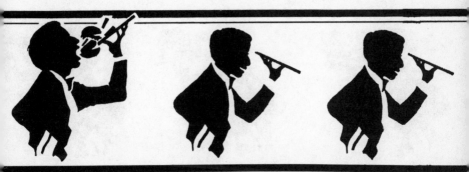

the best there is. (Hold your horses. The author welcomes opposing viewpoints. See WHERE I PIGGED OUT, p. 155).

LOU MITCHELL'S
565 W. Jackson
Chicago, IL

It looks more or less like a hundred other coffee shops—a winding counter, a roomful of tables, a line of customers waiting—but you never had it so good. This just may be the best spot for breakfast in the country. It's certainly the most reliable, with huge portions of extraordinary food at exceptionally reasonable prices: omelets like soufflés, bacon perfectly crisp, pancakes thin and light, and orange juice—the real stuff. Still, it's hell having to order one thing and turn down all the delicious-looking dishes you see on nearby tables. Did I tell you about the double-yolk fried eggs? The wonderful Greek toast? The homemade marmalade? The incredible raisin toast? The perfect waffles? Ecstasy. But Lou Mitchell's would score pigging points if only for the fact that female customers are presented with a complimentary box of Milk Duds the second they walk through the door. I'm tempted to cry "Chauvinism!"—but that's a complaint coming from a man who just might be more interested in free candy than social causes.

REEVES RESTAURANT AND BAKERY
1209 F Street, N.W.
Washington, D.C.

Located amid the glass office buildings and bureaucratic blues

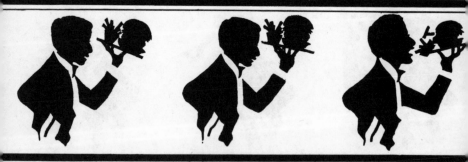

of downtown, this century-old restaurant is a breath of fresh air; in the face of progress, it remains blessedly unchanged. As you enter, you might think your grandmother is in the kitchen: The first sight is of fresh baked goods in display cases laid end-to-end, a chorus line of rolls, doughnuts, cookies, pies, and cakes. (As near to perfect as you get. See also WHERE TO PIG OUT: The Hole Truth and WHERE TO PIG OUT: The Best of the Rest/Best Pie.) Straight ahead, half-block-long wooden counters, flanked by stools, line the walls; a handful of tables lie farther on. Lots of people came here as kids and they keep on coming back. They come for the old-fashioned chicken salad sandwiches, for the homemade mayonnaise, for the fried chicken, spaghetti, and roast-beef specials, for the

world's best strawberry pie. And for the feeling of worn comfort: beveled mirrors, walnut paneling, Tiffany lamps. They don't make them like this anymore.

THE WOMAN'S INDUSTRIAL EXCHANGE
333 N. Charles Street
Baltimore, MD

What started as a small store in the late 1800's, where women in need of money could take their handmade quilts and homemade baked goods and have them sold anonymously, still serves that purpose today. But the shopping can wait; head straight through the salesroom that fronts the street to the tearoom that sits in the back. Yes, tearoom: an unpretentious black-and-white-tiled breakfast and lunching place

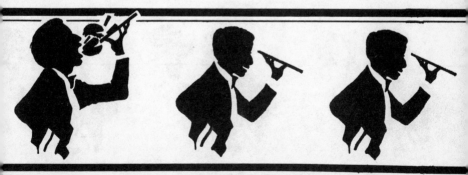

where it is simply impossible to get a bad meal. Piggers depend on its buckwheat cakes, kidney stew, fried oysters, chicken salad (with the obligatory fresh mayonnaise), and devil's-food chocolate cake. Gone are the finger bowls and the silver serving trays, but what's important still remains. Not just top-quality food, but waitresses in delft-blue uniforms, all tearoom veterans, bustling about. Somehow they manage to make you feel like you're the only customer they've got. A classic.

ZABAR'S
2245 Broadway (at 80th Street) New York, NY

Since its humble beginnings as a combination grocery-delicatessen and neighborhood takeout joint, this West Side institution has expanded twice, and though hole-in-the-wall intimacy has given way to industry, every nook, cranny, shelf, and counter is still crammed full and piled high, overflowing with more goodies per square inch than any other place in the country. Where else, in addition to all the traditional deli items, can you find ninety different carry-out dishes, over three hundred cheeses, endless cakes and cookies, prepared meats and salads, smoked fish, fresh-baked breads, Côte Basque pastries, imported chocolates, and homemade pasta? Beats me. But when I die, I hope heaven looks like Zabar's.

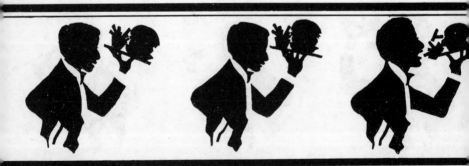

(tie) SONNY BRYAN's
2202 Inwood Road
Dallas, TX

(tie) ANGELO'S
2533 White Settlement Road
Fort Worth, TX

Looking like a fifties roadside stand that was deserted and left for dead, there are no tables at Sonny Bryan's, just twenty-four individual seats with school desktops to rest your elbows on. The sliced beef sandwich reaches an all-time pigging high (see also WHERE TO PIG OUT: Best Bets/The Sandwich Hall of Fame), so unbelievable you'll probably want a second. The homemade onion rings you should order with it are the size of Michelin tires. Bryan's closes up shop as soon as the meat's all gone—anywhere between 4:00 and 7:00 P.M. Which is okay, actually, since this will give you time to jump in the car and head to Fort Worth, where at Angelo's they don't even begin to bring out the ribs until sometime after 5:00. Hidden in an industrial offshoot of downtown, this warehouselike restaurant (windowless, with sawdust on the floor) serves up hickory smoked ribs that—oh, there is a God—match your deepest pigging fantasies: smoky, crusty, and aromatic; tender, meaty, and bursting with flavor. Side orders—potato salad, beans, and especially the coleslaw—stand on their own. All of it together will make you want to stand up and cheer.

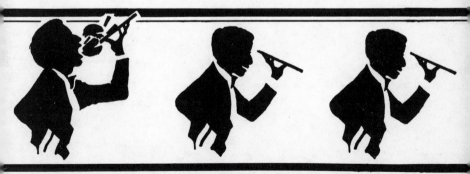

PART IV

WHO PIGS OUT

WHEN THE GOING
GETS TOUGH,
THE TOUGH PIG OUT...

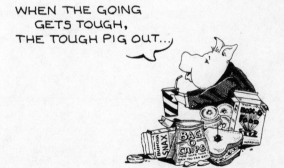

igs don't really pig out. Their diet consists of a concentrated mixture of vegetable products, cornmeal, and soy meal—also known as "sow chow"—which is nondigestible and carried as fat. While basically vegetarians, pigs will eat a little of everything, from insects to leaves to small animals to acorns.

But the platypus—now, *there's* a pigger. Perhaps ounce for ounce the biggest eater in the animal kingdom, this five-pound mammal is able to consume well over its own weight in food. And never gain an ounce.

I hate him.

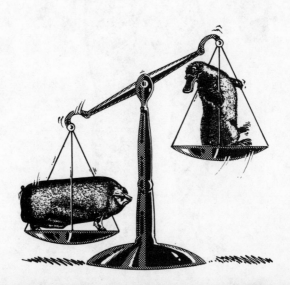

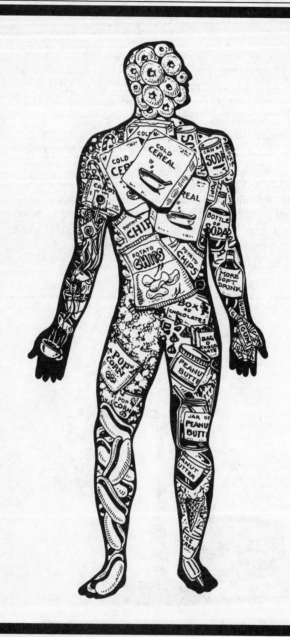

YOU ARE WHAT YOU EAT

During the course of a year, the average American consumes 30 quarts of popcorn, 200 sticks of gum, 17 pounds of candy, another 15 pounds of chocolate, 378 cans of soda, 92 hot dogs, 42 doughnuts, 18 boxes of cold cereal, 14 bags of potato chips, 6 jars of peanut butter, 100 single scoops of ice cream, and 1,217 cups of coffee.

When at a candy machine, the average American will most likely go for a Snickers, unless he or she is from the Northeast, in which case it'll probably be Reese's Peanut Butter Cups.

When the average American goes out to eat, it is usually at a fast-food hamburger place, followed by (in order) a pizza parlor, a fine dining establishment, a seafood restaurant, and a steakhouse. The single most commonly ordered food is a salad; when it comes time for dessert, what is most frequently requested is vanilla ice cream.

IN ANY GIVEN 24 HOURS

Hershey puts out 25 million chocolate Kisses.

Famous Amos bakes 10,000 pounds of cookies.

Kentucky Fried Chicken sells over 2 million 3-piece dinners.

McDonald's does $19,265,000 in business.

Goelitz Confectionery yields 200,000 pounds of Jelly Bellys.

Tootsie Industries makes 10 million Tootsie Rolls.

IHOP customers use 9,315 gallons of syrup (on their 300,175 pancakes).

Nestlé produces 235 million chocolate chips.

THE LAST SUPPER

Q: If you were to die tomorrow, what would your last meal be, where would you eat it, and whom would you share it with?

Erma Bombeck

A: Long—about sixteen courses. In my mom's kitchen. I'd share it with someone who is on a papaya-Perrier diet.

Dr. Joyce Brothers

A: Cottage cheese, so I'd die thin. At Lutèce (what the hell??). My husband, so he'd see how cute I looked before I went.

Stephen King

A: I would first want to have White Castle cheeseburgers for lunch with Kirby McCauley (my friend and agent), followed by a rack of lamb for dinner with my wife, Tabby. I'd like the rack of lamb from Petite Marmite in New York City.

Judith Martin

A: On Miss Manners' dying day, she may indulge in four, rather than her usual three, cucumber sandwiches (one-inch square each), but she will certainly not alter her habit of taking them with a cup of tea, in her own library, with those from her circle of family and friends who are kind enough to stop by. Although she does favor lemon sherbet, she would not consider the occasion sufficient excuse for the barbarity of introducing it at the tea table.

Liz Smith

A: My last meal would be chicken-fried steak, cream gravy, hot biscuits, collard greens, black-eyed peas, creamed carrots, iced tea, pineapple and lettuce salad, and lemon meringue pie . . . [at] The Pink Tea Cup luncheonette on Bleecker Street . . . the greatest for soul food in New York.

Jim Davis, creator of Garfield

A: I love to pig out as much as or more than any other human being . . . my favorite ice cream is mint chip, with chips the size of babies . . . [but] I would start my last meal with a frosty, cold bottle of Dom Pérignon '63, fresh Gulf shrimp with my secret tartar sauce, followed by a strawberry-and-onion salad marinated in a sweet-vinegar dressing. For an entree, I would have blood-rare steak au poivre with the green peppercorns, so as not to overpower the Château Margaux '45. For dessert, I should think the Château d'Yquem would be best, accompanied by a bowl of fresh blueberries. And as long as we are dreaming here, I would top the meal off with a hot steaming cauldron of King Louis XV cognac and a big, black Cuban cigar. I would have the meal in the bar of the Helmsley Palace with all my friends in attendance.

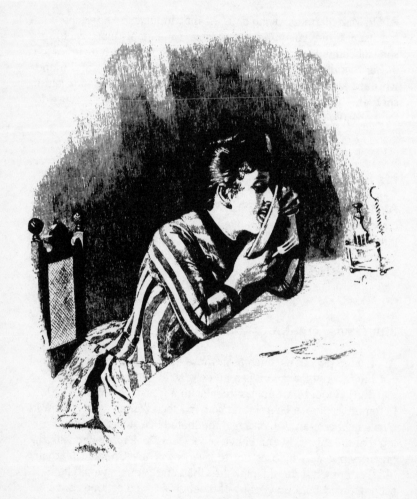

WHO PIGS OUT

SECRET VICES, GUILTY PLEASURES

A look at some well-known people and their little-known favorite indulgences:

DAN RATHER . . . . Fudgsicles

NEIL SIMON. . . . . popcorn

ANN LANDERS . . . . chocolate

WILLIAM F. BUCKLEY. . . . . peanut butter

GOLDA MEIR. . . . . Häagen-Dazs vanilla ice cream

HELEN GURLEY BROWN. . . . . . waffles

MARY TYLER MOORE . . . . bubble gum

MARLENE DIETRICH . . . . hot dogs

DR. JOYCE BROTHERS . . . . chocolate-covered marshmallows

ERMA BOMBECK. . . . . pasta

GLORIA STEINEM . . . . Sara Lee and anything from a machine

JUDITH MARTIN. . . . . "Miss Manners admits of neither vices nor addictions. If she has secrets, it is because she does not tell them."

OUT OF ORDER

The average person consumes close to 160 candy bars a year, but are you so busy eating them that you haven't taken time to notice how really beautiful they are? Opposite is a quiz to test this possible pigging oversight. Advanced piggers who have proven themselves able to eat M & M's while blindfolded—and still identify the color of each—may be excused. Otherwise, name, if you can, the candy bars from which the following cross-sections have been cut.

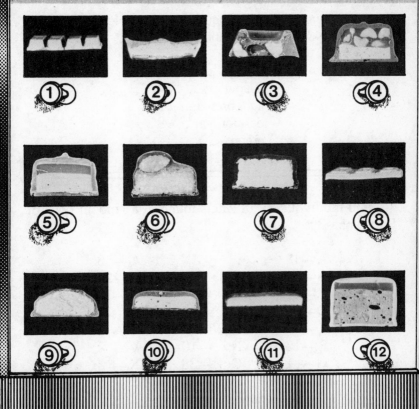

OUT OF ORDER: Candy Quiz

Ten, Nine, Eight, Seven, Six . . .

For the curious pigger, the frequency of colors found in a sample bag of M & M's (half-pound size) . . .

orange 62
yellow 54
light brown 32
dark brown 98
green 17

. . . and the frequency of letters found in a random bowl of Post Alpha-Bits.*

A—18	I — 7	Q— 8
B—59	J — 2	R—24
C— 1	K — 4	S—11
D—35	L —11	T— 2
E—10	M/W— 5	U— 1
F—16	N/Z —10	V— 2
G— 1	O —38	X— 2
H—19	P —25	Y—15

Broken/Indistinguishable—17

*Alpha-Bits are what piggers call "food for thought." Before consumption, numerous word games can be played. With a discreet nibble, Scrabble is made easy: E's become F's, Q's turn into O's, R's can be made into P's.

STUDENT PIGGING

An Oral Report

In 1976, the Benton, Arkansas, senior high school was losing $1,000 a month on its student hot-lunch program when it decided to turn the cafeteria into a McDonald's franchise. The menu offered traditional McDonald's fare with the exception of the milk shake, which school officials vetoed in order to get students to drink federally financed milk. Not that it made a difference. The number of students buying lunch rose dramatically, from ten to over sixty percent. The only parental complaint came from a mother who asked that the cafeteria not serve McDonald's food for lunch because that was what she always served her kids for dinner.

Whether Benton High graduates who go on to college are most likely to attend the University of Cincinnati, Ohio State, and DePaul University—all of which house a McDonald's on campus—has yet to be determined. But graduates choosing to join the U.S. military should be interested to know that at the Naval Exchange on the base in Pearl Harbor, a Burger King franchise has replaced a cafeteria-style food-service operation.

Likewise, student piggers seeking a more specialized academic program might try making the grade at Carvel College (also known as Sundae School), at BKU (that's Burger King University), or at Hamburger University. The latter, like the United Nations, is equipped with simultaneous translation and offers classes in the correct way to fold a Big Mac box, how to put out a shortening fire (dump frozen French fries on it), and carbonation principles. Graduates receive a "Bachelor of Hamburgerology" degree—with a minor in fries.

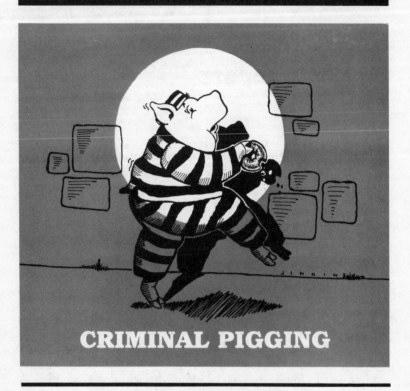

CRIMINAL PIGGING

Anything You Eat
Can and Will
Be Used Against You

Proof, beyond a reasonable doubt, that food—not love—can drive a normal person to extremes.

In 1933, Bonnie Parker and Clyde Barrow held up the First Bank of Stanfield, Kansas. The two escaped with $27,500 in cash and a recipe for caramel corn that had been safeguarded in the bank's vault for seven generations.

In 1956, Noel Carriou got so mad when his wife made the roast beef too rare that during a heated argument after dinner, he literally kicked her out of bed with such force that she fell to the floor, broke her neck, and died. After serving a seven-year prison sentence, Carriou was released and subsequently married again. One evening, Clemence, his second wife, mistakenly *burnt* the roast. In a tirade, Carriou picked up a kitchen knife and, complaining that she cooked "like a Nazi," proceeded to stab her to death. A French jury, perhaps sympathetic to one man's passion for good food, sentenced him to only eight years behind bars.

In 1979, Dan White was convicted of manslaughter for the slayings of San Francisco Mayor George Moscone and Supervisor Harvey Milk. His attorney, Doug Schmidt, pleaded the "Twinkie Defense," contending that White had pigged out on Hostess Twinkies, and that the sugary ingredients had caused diminished capacity to judge right and wrong.

In 1981, Cornelius Jefferson hijacked a delivery truck in Houston, Texas. His take? Thirty thousand dollars' worth of salami, Swiss cheese, okra, and cherry pie.

Later in 1981, James Sims, a cook, and Angela Robinson, a waitress, perpetrated "The Great Cookie Caper," and attempted to sell the secret recipes for Mother's Cookies to the bakers at Pepperidge Farm for a cool $24,000 per dozen. It wasn't difficult for authorities to track down the criminals—the anonymous extortion letter had a return address on it—and Sims and Robinson were arrested and charged with possession of stolen property and selling of trade secrets.

The defense rests.

In October, 1982, John DeLorean, the automobile manufacturer, was arrested and charged with conspiracy to sell cocaine. His first words to his wife, Cristina, after being released on $10 million bail: "I want a hamburger."

THE PIGGER HALL OF FAME

Admission to the Pigger Hall of Fame is a distinguished honor bestowed upon a select few whose example, either daily or on a given occasion, has taught and inspired; whose contributions have made pigging not only a way of life, but a reflection of life.

In the chips

Wally Amos. Founder, the Famous Amos Chocolate Chip Cookie. He put chic into chips, turned an American tradition into a superstar, and introduced a commercially available c.c.c. that didn't taste like sawdust.

I'm just a guy who can't say no . . .

Diamond Jim Brady. Multimillionaire railroad baron. Described by a New York restauranteur as "the best twenty-five customers I ever had." Dinner alone included three dozen oysters, six crabs, several bowls of turtle soup, half a dozen lobsters, a pair of ducks, a double serving of terrapin, a sirloin steak, vegetables, and a few gallons of orange juice, his favorite drink. Dessert amounted to a platter of pies and cakes, and two pounds of candy.

He died on a sundae

J. Ackerman Coles. Physician, art collector. Numerous real estate holdings. Upon his death, his will left a trust fund to the city of Scotch Plains, New Jersey, stipulating that the kids who lived there be treated to free ice cream once a year.

A good deal, yes, but no one should have to listen to his commercials

Tom Carvel. Owner, Carvel Ice Cream. In 1937, his business became the first anywhere to introduce the "buy one, get one free" marketing concept.

He did it all for you

Jim Delligatti. McDonald's franchisee, Pittsburgh, Pennsylvania. Invented the Big Mac after losing sales to a nearby competitor who sold big sandwich-style hamburgers. He is credited by the company for his idea, but other than aiding his own business, he received no royalty or compensation.

Eat one a day and call me in the morning

Nathan Handwerker. Proprieter, Nathan's hot dogs. Angered the competition by selling franks for a nickel when everyone else was charging a dime. To counteract their rumors that he was using dog- or horsemeat and could thereby charge less, Handwerker called on a friend whose son was a doctor. That afternoon, dressed in lab coats and with stethoscopes around their necks, a quartet of medicos stood outside his store, wolfing down hot dogs. Word got around that doctors were eating at Nathan's, and business flourished.

Let them eat fries

Tom Kavano and Reenie Palmiere. Married in 1975. The ceremony was formal, but the reception was held under the golden arches of a Westmont, New Jersey, McDonald's. The menu included Big Mac cake and champagne.

Surprise, Surprise, Surprise!

Wendy Potasnik. Age 9. Filed suit against the Cracker Jack Division of Borden, Inc., claiming false advertising and breach of contract because a box she bought failed to contain a toy surprise. She later agreed to drop the suit after she received a letter of apology and a coupon for a free box.

Never too late

Harland Sanders. Kentucky Colonel. Began franchising his regionally famous fried-chicken recipe in 1956, when he was a sixty-six-year-old, $105-a-month beneficiary of Social Security. Today, the "little business" he started grosses over $2.3 billion a year, has 655 stores in 48 countries, and sells 200 million pieces of chicken a month.

A meal so good you could die

Milton Schapp. Former governor of Pennsylvania. In 1976, he attempted to negate bad publicity by eating lunch at Philadelphia's Bellevue Stratford, site of the ill-fated American Legion convention.

La pièce de résistance

Francois Vatel. Chef. In the late seventeenth century, he committed suicide over a meal that did not turn out to be what was expected.

Give a guy a brake

Pigger unknown. A Frenchman. Able to digest one and a half pounds of metal a day. In March 1982, over a fifteen-day period, he ate a ten-speed bicycle.

HOW SWEET IT IS

How do chocoholics remove melted chocolate from their hands? A few (2.5 percent) use a dry cloth; a sensible 25.3 percent use a wet cloth, but a smart 65.3 percent use their tongues.

This is just one of the chocolate eating habits examined in a survey conducted by The Nestlé Company of 285 chocolate lovers attending a 1982 chocolate fair in Chicago.

According to the survey, 22 percent have their first bite of chocolate before breakfast; 43.5 percent have something chocolate at or after dinner; and almost all (87.9 percent) binge again before bedtime.

One respondent wrote, "I always keep an emergency chocolate bar behind the chicken in the freezer, one in my desk at work, and one in the car for commuting."

Milk chocolate was preferred by 48.7 percent of the participants, semi-sweet by 42.6 percent, and white chocolate by a select 4.6 percent.

"What goes best with chocolate?" Anything from milk (23.5 percent) and ice cream (19.4 percent), to beer (1.2 percent), friends (6.7 percent), "everything" (11.1 percent), "nothing" (2 percent), and— what else?—more chocolate (8.3 percent).

"Have you ever tried to give up chocolate?" Only 22.8 percent said yes—reasons being to diet or for Lent. For 21.5 percent of these abstainers, going cold turkey lasted one to three weeks; 4.6 percent held out for less than a day.

"How does eating so much chocolate make you feel?" A total of 38.9 percent replied "indulgent," 19.3 percent admitted "guilty," 12.3 percent said "decadent," 12.3 percent confessed "titillated," and 4.2 answered "philosophical."

"GIVE ME CHOCOLATE—OR GIVE ME DEATH": ARE YOU A CHOCOHOLIC?

YES   NO

1. Forget "career vs. relationship"; for you, is a *major* decision having to choose between white and dark, milk and bittersweet, with almonds and without?

2. Is the fastest way to get your attention the mere mention of the words *free samples*?

3. Do you look at vanilla as somebody's idea of a joke?

4. Would you campaign to have Sara Lee's birthday declared a national holiday?

5. Has an M & M never had enough time to melt in your hands?

6. Have you mastered the art of sucking the middle from inside a malted-milk ball and still leaving the outer coating intact?

7. Is your most frequent form of daily exercise prying off the lid from a container of Häagen-Dazs chocolate chocolate chip?

8. Do you consider Ding Dongs one of mankind's most significant cultural achievements?

9. Have you ever eaten an entire box of *still-frozen* brownies because you were unable to wait long enough for them to thaw?

10. Is your ulterior motive for visiting sick friends to pick through the boxes of candies they've received?

11. Did it come as a surprise to you that Bill Blass also designed clothes?

12. Are you of the conviction that Famous Amos should be made a patron saint?

13. Does "dinner with a few intimate friends" really mean Godiva, Teuscher, Cadbury, and Krön?

14. Is your idea of foreplay a bag of Hershey's Kisses?

15. Do you consider carob a Communist plot?

If you have answered yes to any one of these questions, there is definite warning that you may be a chocoholic.

If you have answered yes to any two, the chances are that you are a chocoholic.

If you have answered yes to three or more, wipe your face.

PART V

WE CAN'T GO ON EATING LIKE THIS . . .

CAUGHT WITH YOUR HAND IN THE COOKIE JAR: THE OFFICIAL PIGGER'S EXCUSE LISTS

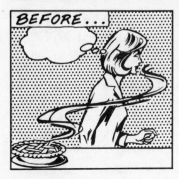

IT'S A HOLIDAY.
I'M ON VACATION.
I DESERVE IT.
IT'S NOT FATTENING.
I JUST EXERCISED.
I'VE BEEN DEPRESSED.
IT'S HEALTH FOOD.
SOMEONE WENT TO A LOT OF TROUBLE.
PEOPLE ARE STARVING IN . . .

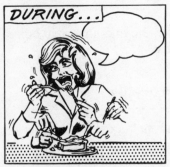

IT WOULD HAVE GONE TO WASTE.
I DIDN'T WANT TO THROW IT AWAY.
I FELT FAINT.
I NEEDED THE PROTEIN.
I'M HAVING AN ANXIETY ATTACK.
I HAVEN'T EATEN ALL DAY.
I NEVER TRIED THIS BEFORE.
IT SMELLED SO GOOD.
I COULDN'T CONTROL MYSELF.

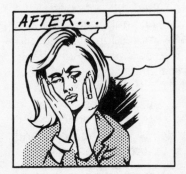

I FORGOT.
I ONLY ATE THE BROKEN ONES.
I BARELY TOUCHED IT.
I DIDN'T SWALLOW.
I WAS JUST NIBBLING.
I ONLY WANTED A TASTE.
I ONLY HAD A LITTLE.
I DIDN'T EAT IT ALL.
I'M STARTING MY DIET TOMORROW.

DRESS FOR EXCESS

hat's the joy of pigging out if you're going to be in total agony while you're doing it? Sitting down to ribs at Angelo's in that tight pair of jeans may not appear to be a problem, but try standing up when you're finished and you could be in for trouble.

Clothes are as important a part of pigging out as the perfect hamburger, the proper etiquette, and the appropriate excuse. A pigger's wardrobe must satisfy three basic requirements:

PRACTICALITY

Pig-out clothes must be sensible. White and pastels are best avoided; black and dark colors are wisest, as they will not show stains, dribbles, spots, or other telltale signs. Likewise, all fabrics should be Scotchgarded so they can be wiped clean with a damp cloth.

Large pockets come strongly recommended. They not only free hands, but provide sufficient storage space for stealing complimentary hors d'oeuvres, taking leftovers, and sneaking extra helpings from the one-time-only buffet table.

COMFORT

The main goal of dressing for excess is to be as comfortable as possible. Belt is a four-letter word. It constricts the stomach and can cause a false impression of being full.

Elastic and expandable waistbands are obvious choices. Likewise, sweats, tunics, and caftans. Cotton is the preferred fabric, as it stretches with the body and allows it to breathe.

DEFENSIVE DRESSING

Piggers never know when vanity might set in. For that reason alone, black serves a special purpose, enabling you to look slim despite the massive amounts of potatoes, rolls, and chocolate cheesecake you've consumed. Checkered clothes can also work in the pigger's favor, as others will find it difficult to tell where your stomach ends and the tablecloth begins.

The closest you should ever come to horizontal stripes is a seven-layer cake.

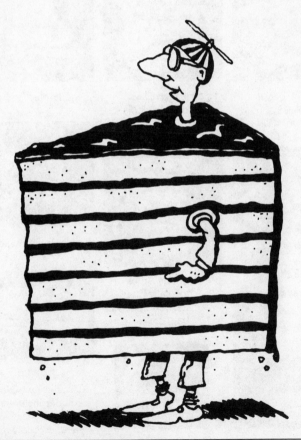

THE LAST GREAT CALORIE GUIDE

Forget the hard-boiled eggs. Never mind the cottage cheese. For the weight-conscious pigger, the complete lowdown on the really *important* foods:

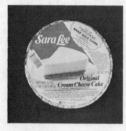

Sara Lee Cheesecake original 1380 for two 834

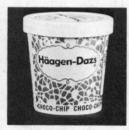

Häagen-Dazs chocolate chocolate chip (pint) 1,236

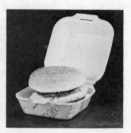

Big Mac 563

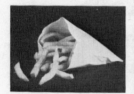

French fries (McDonald's, regular) 220

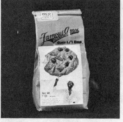

Famous Amos Chocolate Chip Cookies (one-pound bag) 1,840

Jelly Belly 3 each

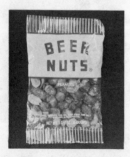

Beer Nuts 167/oz.

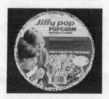

Jiffy Pop 630/pan

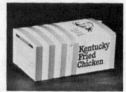

Kentucky Fried Chicken (two-piece dinner including mashed potatoes, gravy, coleslaw, and roll) 661

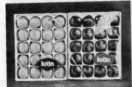

Krön chocolate
dark 78/oz.
milk 110/oz.

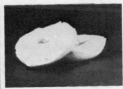

Bagel with cream
cheese 265

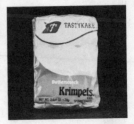

Tastykake Butterscotch
Krimpets (one pkg.)
195

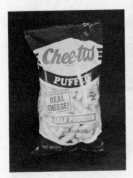

Chee-Tos 160/oz.

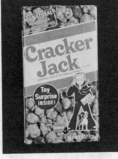

Cracker Jack 120/oz.

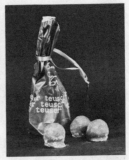

Teuscher champagne
truffles 200 each

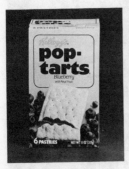

Pop-Tarts 210 each

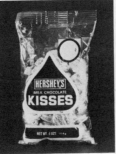

Hershey Kisses 25
each

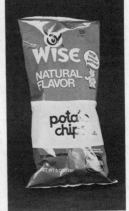

Wise Potato Chips
160/oz.

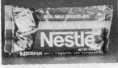

Nestlé milk chocolate
morsels 3 each

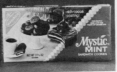

Mystic Mint 88 each

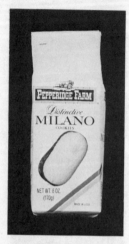

Milano 63 each

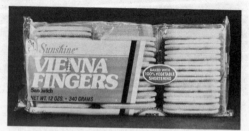

Sunshine Vienna Finger 71 each

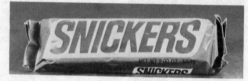

Snickers (two-oz. bar) 270

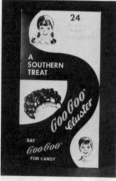

Goo Goo Clusters 245 each

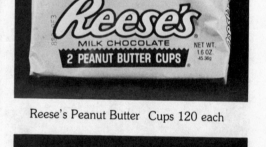

Reese's Peanut Butter Cups 120 each

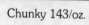

Chunky 143/oz.

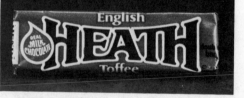

Heath (1$\frac{1}{8}$-oz. bar) 170

WE CAN'T GO ON EATING LIKE THIS

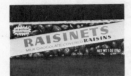
Raisinets 115/oz.

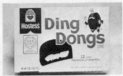
Ding Dong 170 each

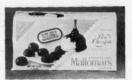
Mallomar 55 each

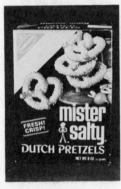
Mr. Salty
Pretzels110/oz.

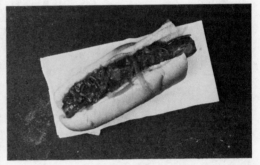
Hot Dog
(with mustard, relish, onions) 345

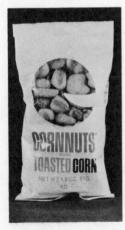
Corn Nuts 130/oz.

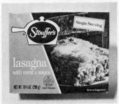
Stouffer's Lasagna 770

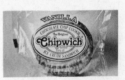
Chipwich 290 each

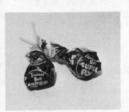
Tootsie Roll Pops
48 each

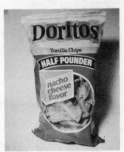
Doritos 140/oz.

THE PIGGER'S 21-DAY DIET

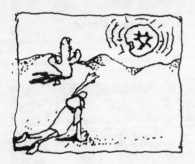

Daily Intake: 1,000 Calories (Give or Take a Few)

Day 1: 7 Twinkies

Day 2: 235 M & M's (plain)

Day 3: 83 Animal Crackers

Day 4: ½ package raw Pillsbury chocolate-chip cookie dough

Day 5: 3 loaves Stouffer's French bread pizza (cheese)

Day 6: 6 glazed doughtnuts

Day 7: 20 Oreos

Day 8: 111 Life Savers

WE CAN'T GO ON EATING LIKE THIS

Day   9:   5 White Castle cheeseburgers

Day 10:   40 marshmallows

Day 11:   200 Fritos

Day 12:   10 Fudgsicles

Day 13:   8 Kentucky Fried Chicken drumsticks
(or 7 wings/5 breasts/4 thighs)

Day 14:   9 Dairy Queen ice-cream cones (small)

Day 15:   48 Triscuits

Day 16: $4\frac{1}{2}$ Thomas' English Muffins (buttered)

Day 17:   250 Reese's pieces

Day 18:   8 frozen waffles

Day 19:   2 Quarter Pounders with cheese

Day 20:   28 Kraft caramels

Day 21:   91 malted-milk balls

R.I.P.
Gone but Not Forgotten

Red M & M's. Long the favorite of many, production was discontinued in March 1976, with the governmental ban on red dye #2. The M & M/Mars Candy Company made up for the loss by increasing the number of green and introducing a new color, orange.

Fizzies. Grape-, cola-, cherry-, orange-, and lemon-lime-flavored tablets that when dropped in water did just what their name promised and produced a glass of soda. More adventurous piggers used to drop them directly into their mouths and then rush to the bathroom mirror to watch.

The Hula Burger. A little-known and less successful McDonald's menu offering (it included pineapple and cheese on a bun) that disappeared by the mid-1970's, but to this day remains founder Ray Kroc's personal favorite.

Flav-R-Straws. They looked like ordinary drinking straws, but the insides contained either chocolate or strawberry "mixes"; hence, as you drank your milk through them, it automatically got flavored.

Pop Rocks. Available only for a limited time (1977–78) in limited distribution, General Foods introduced this candy craze where a crystallized powder was poured from a packet onto the tongue and the explosive result had to be experienced to be believed.

Girl Scout Mint Cookies. Included in this group due to technical error. The Girl Scouts still sell cookies and they still have the mint ones. But let's be honest. They just aren't the same as they once were—and sorry, kids, they just don't taste as good.

Attention nostalgic piggers: Atomic fireballs, button candies, licorice pipes, pixie sticks—all those childhood treats you thought were long gone—are still available and marketed. See WHERE TO PIG OUT: The Best of the Rest-/Best Penny Candy Selection.

WHERE I PIGGED OUT

Obviously I couldn't get everywhere. So let me know about the pig-out spots I missed and any other restaurant worth mentioning, if only for one particular food or special deal offer.

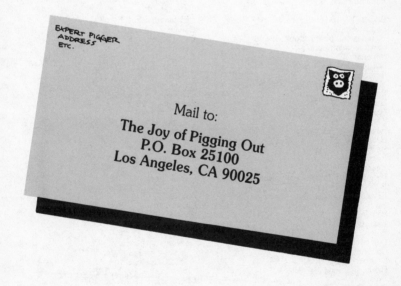

EXPERT PIGGER
ADDRESS
ETC.

Mail to:

The Joy of Pigging Out
P.O. Box 25100
Los Angeles, CA 90025

If you include your name and address and I use your suggestion in a future book, I'll send you a free copy.

Note: Specific restaurants are listed in the Geographical Index.

GENERAL INDEX

A & W Rootbeer, 10, 96
All you can eat, 76–77
Almond Joy, 131
Alpha-Bits, 132
Amighetti special sandwich, 47
Amos, Wally, 136
Amusement park food, 87
Angel-food cake, 41
Animal Crackers, 10, 152
Appetizer, most unusual, 70
Apple pie, 24, 73, 82
Apples, 29
Atomic fireballs, 154
Auteuils, 45
Automats, 103

Baba au rhum, 45
Baby Ruth, 8
Bagels, 17, 102, 149
Baguettes, 47
Bakeries and pastry shops, 45–48
Banana cream pie, 73
Bananas, 29
Bar Mitzvahs, 85
Barbecoa, 100
Barbecue guide to Texas, 100–101
Barbecued ribs, 17, 21
Barrow, Clyde, 134
Basic food groups, 15–17
Baskin-Robbins, 10
Beach foods, 86
Bear claws, 17
Beer nuts, 17, 148
Beignets, 31
Belgian waffles, 17
Betty Crocker factory tour (Minneapolis), 93
Big Mac (McDonald's), 11, 137, 148
Black-eyed peas, 105
Blass, Bill, 141
Blintzes, 102
Blue food, 20
Blueberry doughnuts, 38
Bombeck, Erma, 126, 129
Bonbons, 17, 87
Bourbon balls, 30–31
Brady, Diamond Jim, 136
Bread, 17
    bagels, 17, 102, 149
    bakeries and pastry shops, 45–48
    English muffins, 10, 17
    pumpernickel, 8
    rye, 17, 102
    sourdough, 17, 46
    white, 28–29
Bread pudding, 75
Breakfast guide, 80–82
Brie, 17
Brothers, Joyce, 126, 129

Brown, Helen Gurley, 129
Brownies, 17
Bryant, Arthur, 111
Bubble gum, 129
Buckley, William F., 129
Buffalo chicken wings, 111
Burger King, 11, 133
Burger King University, 133
Butter, 28
Butterfingers, 131
Button candy, 154

Cadbury, 141
Cafeterias, 40–41
Cakes, 17
    cheesecakes, 3, 10, 17, 21, 30, 102
    chocolate, 74
    Drake's, 27
    Entenmann's, 27
Calorie guide, 148–151
Canapés, 85
Candy apples, 87
Candy bars, 17
    calorie guide to, 150–151
    recognition quiz for, 131
Candy canes, 23
Candy eating contests, 89
Candygram, 29
Cannoli, 17, 45
Caramel corn, 17, 134
Caramels, 31
    Kraft, 153
Carnival food, 87
Carriou, Noel, 135
Carrot cake, 41
Carvel, Tom, 137
Carvel College, 133
Caviar, 17, 85
Celery, 29
Challah French toast, 102
Charcuterie, 41, 84
Cheese dogs, 17
Cheesecake, 21
    Junior's mail-ordered, 30, 102
    Miss Grimble, 102
    Sara Lee, 3, 10, 17, 148
Cheesesteak, 17, 67, 86. 107
Chee-Tos, 17, 149
Chicago deep-dish pizza guide, 110
Chicago food festival, 94
Chicken, 111
    delivery of, 29
    Kentucky Fried, 125, 138, 148, 153
Chicken-fried steak, 41
Chicken liver, 77
Chicken-pan pie, 105
Chiles rellenos, 101

Chili, 101, 111
Chili dogs, 17, 39
Chinese food, 17
    delivery of, 29
    of San Francisco, 109
Chinese roast pork sandwich, 68
Chipwich, 151
Chocolate, 24, 129, 139
    chocoholic test, 140–141
    Hershey, 6, 92–93
    Krön, 93, 141, 149
    most unusual, 70
    Nestlé, 7, 125, 139
Chocolate bunnies, 24
Chocolate cake, best, 74
Chocolate caramels, 31, 47
Chocolate chip cookies, 82
    David's, 11, 17, 65, 76
    Famous Amos, 11, 17, 125, 136, 141, 148
    Toll House, 7
Chocolate-covered doughnuts, 37
Chocolate-covered marshmallows, 129
Chocolate cream pie, 73
Chocolate Orgasm, 46
Chocolate pudding, 21
Chocolate split, 41
Chopped liver, 17, 102
Christmas food, 23
Chunky, 131, 150
Cinnamon, 29
Cinnamon-covered graham crackers, 17
Cinnamon rolls, 17, 46
Clothing, 146–147
Cincinnati chili, 111
Coca-Cola, 10, 42
Cocoa mix, 29
Coconut-flaked doughnuts, 37
Coffee, 82
Coffee shops, 35
    best office buildings, 74
Cold food, 20
Cold salads, 41
Coles, J. Ackerman, 136
Combination dinner, most unusual, 70
Contests, food-eating, 89–90
Continental Baking Company, 7
Cookies, 17, 93
    Animal Crackers, 10, 152
    best, 64–65
    David's, 11, 17, 65, 76
    Famous Amos, 11, 17, 125, 136, 141, 148
    Girl Scout, 154
    Hydrox and Oreo, 9
    Lorna Doone, 9
    Milano, 17, 21, 22, 65, 150
    Mystic Mint, 17, 65, 149
    opening a bag of Pepperidge Farm, 22
    See also Chocolate chip cookies
Corn dogs, 39
Corn nuts, 12, 151
Cotton candy, 87
Country-fried steak, 105
Crabs, 77
Cracker Jack, 10, 17, 87, 138, 149
Cream cheese, 29
Cream-filled doughnuts, 37
Creighton, Emma, 91
Croissants, 17

Croutons, 29
Crum, George, 5
Crumpets, 17
Cuban sandwich, 68
Cupcakes, 45

Dairy Queen, 10, 153
David's Cookies, 11, 17, 65, 76
Davis, Jim, 127
Deep-dish pizza, 110
Delancey St. Delicatessen (New York City), 10
Delligatti, Jim, 137
DeLorean, John, 135
Desserts, best homemade, 72–73
Devil Dogs, 17
Dewar, Jimmy, 7
Dietrich, Marlene, 129
"Diner," 35
Ding Dongs, 17, 140, 151
Dinner Rolls, 47
Dorgan, Ted, 9
Doritos, 151
Doughnuts, 152
    best bets for, 37–38
    jelly, 21
    Krispy Kreme, 27
Down-home cooking guide, 105–107
Drake's Cakes, 27

Easter, 24
"EAT," 35
Eclairs, 17, 45
Egg cream, 103
Egg rolls, 72
Eggnog, 23
English muffins, 10, 17
Entenmann's, 27
Epperson, Frank, 7
Eskimo Pies, 17
Ethnic food festivals, 94–95
Etiquette, 18–20

Factory tours, 92–93
Falaffel, 84
Familiar food group, 16–17
Famous Amos Chocolate Chip Cookies, 11,
    17, 125, 136, 141, 148
Fast food group, 16–17
Feast of San Gennaro (New York City), 95
Ferdi special sandwich, 67
Feuchtwanger, Anton, 6–7
Finest food group, 16–17
Fish 'n' chips, 17
Fizzies, 154
Flav-R-Straws, 154
Food-eating contests, 89–90
Food festivals
    ethnic, 94–95
    most unusual, 71
Food groups, basic, 15–17
Foot-long hot dogs, 17
Foreign food group, 16–17
Fourth of July food, 24
Freed, Julius, 9
Freihoeffer's Cookies, 27
French bread, 17
French fries, 17, 74, 86, 148
French toast, 17

Malted-milk eggs, 24
Malteds, 17
Maple syrup, 4
Marie Antoinette, 4
"Marquise," 47
Mars, Forrest, 7
Mars Candies, 7
Marshmallow chickens, 24
Marshmallow, 17, 153
  chocolate covered, 129
Martin, Judith, 127, 129
McDonald's, 10, 125, 133, 137
Meir, Golda, 129
Memorial Day, 24
Menudo, 100
Meringues, 45
Milano (Pepperidge Farm), 17, 21, 22, 65,
    150
Milk chocolate, 139
Milk shakes, 17, 43, 72
Milky Way, 10, 17, 131
Miss Grimble Cheesecake, 102
Mr. Salty Pretzels, 151
Mrs. Paul's Fish Sticks, 17
Moore, Mary Tyler, 129
Mother's Cookies, 135
Mounds, 10, 131
Movie theaters, 87
Muffuletta, 68
Murrie, Bruce, 7
Mystic Mint Cookies (Nabisco), 17, 65, 149

Nabisco, 9
  New Jersey factory tour of, 93
Name, most unusual restaurant, 70
Napoleons, 17, 45
Necco Wafers, 87
Nestlé Company, 7, 125, 139
Nestlé Milk Chocolate Morsels, 149
Nestlé Quick, 10
New York City, 95
  "Deli" guide to, 102
  old New York Guide, 103
Ninth Avenue International Food Festival
    (New York City), 95
Noodles, 84

Omelets, 41, 43
Operas, 45
Orange Julius, 9
Ore-Ida Tater Tots, 17
Oreo Cookies, 9, 17, 152
Orleans (Pepperidge Farm), 22
Orville Redenbacher's Popcorn, 17
Oyster bars, 85
  best, 74
Oyster eating contest, 90

Palmiere, Reenie, 137
Pancake house, best, 74–75
Pancakes, 17
Parker, Bonnie, 134
Parmesan cheese, 28
Passover, 25
Pasta, 20, 41, 76, 103, 129
Pastrami on rye, 10
Pastry shops and bakeries, 45–48
Pâté, 85

Peanut butter, 6, 28, 29, 129
  Peter Pan, 10
Peanut butter cookies, 47
Peanut butter pocket doughnut, 38
Peanuts, 87
  best, 75
Pecan pie, 73
Penny candy, 154
  best selection of, 72
Pepperidge Farm, 7, 135
  Connecticut factory tour of, 93
  Milano, 17, 21, 22, 65, 150
  opening a bag of, 22
  Orleans, 22
Peter Pan Peanut Butter, 10
Philadelphia street-food guide, 107–108
Picking at food, 19
Pickled herring, 85
Pies, 17
  best, 73
Pigs, 123
Pilgrims, 4
Pillsbury chocolate chip cookies dough, 17, 152
Pittsburgh Folk Festival, 95
Pixie Sticks, 154
Pizza, 20, 21, 103
  Chicago deep-dish, 110
  delivery of, 29
Pizza Hut, 11
Platypus, 123
Plum pudding, 23
Poor Boys, 17, 67
Pop Rocks, 154
Popcorn, 3, 87, 129
  best, 75, 148
Popsicle, 7
Pop-Tarts, 17, 149
Potasnik, Wendy, 138
Potato chips, 3, 5
  Jay's, 27
  Wise, 10, 27, 149
Potato skins, 53
Powdered doughnuts, 37
Presto Pizza, 86
Pretzels, 3
  Mr. Salty, 108
  soft, 108
Prime ribs, 82
Prime ribs hash, 77
Pringles, 17
Prosciutto, 17, 85
Pumpernickel bread, 8
Pumpkin pie, 23
  eating contest, 89

Quarter Pounder, 153

Raisinets, 17, 151
Rather, Dan, 129
Ravioli, 17
"Red hots," 40
Reese, H. B., 6
Reese's Peanut Butter Cup, 6, 21, 125, 131,
    150
Reese's Pieces, 11, 153
Religieuses, 45
Ribs, 111
  barbecued, 17, 21

Rice Krispies Marshmallow Treats, 10
Rich's Bavarian Creme Puffs, 17
Roast beef, 23, 41, 107, 135
Robinson, Angela, 135
Rock Cornish game hen, 84
Rosen's poppy-seed buns, 40
Rosh Hashanah, 25
Rudkin, Margaret, 7
Rye bread, 17, 102

Salami, 31
Salisbury, J. H., 48
Sally Lunn, 45
Salsiccia Pinwheel, 48
Saltwater taffy, 31
San Francisco Oriental food guide, 108–109
Sanders, Harland, 138
Sanders Hot Fudge, 27
Sandwiches, 66–68, 83, 102
   hoagies, 108
Sara Lee, 129, 140
   cheesecake, 3, 10, 17, 148
   Illinois factory tour of, 92
"Saratoga Chips," 5
Schapp, Milton, 138
Seafood, best inexpensive, 74
See's Candies, 27
Semi-sweet chocolate, 139
Service in restaurants, 36
Sewell, Ike, 110
Sfogliatelle, 45
Shish-kebab, 84
Shopping-mall food, 83–84
Shrimp cocktails, 85
Simon, Neil, 129
Sims, James, 135
Sliced-beef sandwich, 67
Sloppy Joe, 67
Smelt eating contest, 90
Smith, Liz, 127
Smithfield Ham, 31
Smorgasbord, 21
Smoked fish, 41
Snickers, 10, 17, 125, 131, 150
Soda fountain, best drugstore, 75
Soft pretzels, 108
Soup, 41, 82
Sourdough bread, 17, 46
Souvlaki, 85
Spaghetti, 17
Special occasions, 85
Spencer, Dee Dee, 91
Splits, 17
Sponge cake, 47
Stadium food, 87
Standard Candy Company factory tour
      (Nashville), 93
Steak, 78–79
Steinem, Gloria, 129
Stevens, Harry, 9
Sticky buns, 17
Stouffer's French Bread Pizza, 152
Stouffer's Lasagna, 17, 151
Strawberry pie, 73
Strawberry waffles, 80
Street vendors, 84
   most unusual, 70
   Sabrett, 39

Stuffed mushrooms, 85
Submarines, 17
Sugar, 29
Sugar cookies, 23
Sugar Pops, 10
Sundaes, 17
   guide to, 58–63
Sunday bread, 47
Sunshine Biscuit Company, 9
Sunshine Vienna Fingers, 150
Sushi, 17
Suzy Q's, 17
   best, 74
Swedish pancakes, 80
Sweet Memories Candy Shop, 89
Sweet potatoes, 17

Tacos, 17, 100–101
Tamales, 17, 100–101
Tarts, 45
Taste of Chicago (food festival), 94
Tastykakes, 17, 27, 149
Telephoning for food, 29
Tempura, 84
Teuscher, 141
Teuscher champagne truffles, 149
Tex-Mex guide to Texas, 100–101
Texas barbecue guide, 99
Thanksgiving food, 23
Theme, most unusual restaurant, 70
Thomas' English Muffins, 10, 153
Three Musketeers, 8
Toast, 28–29
Toasted ravioli, 76
Toll House Cookies, 7
Tootsie Roll, 9, 125
Tootsie Roll Pops, 151
Top ten restaurants, 112–119
Torrone, 45
Tostadas, 17, 100–101
Tours of factories, 92–93
Triscuits, 153
Turkish taffy, 17
Twinkies, 4, 7, 17, 135, 152
Turkey, 23, 41

Unusual food, 69–71
Utensils, 18

Valentine's Day, 24
Van de Kamp's, 27
Vanderbilt, Cornelius, 5
Vanilla, 29
Vatel, Francois, 138
Velveeta Cheese, 10, 17
Vermicelli, 17
Vienna Fingers, 17, 150

Waffles, 129, 153
Waitresses, 36
Wakefield, Ruth, 7
Washington, George, 4
Weddings, 85
White, Dan, 135
White bread, 28–29
White Castle Hamburgers, 30, 153

GEOGRAPHICAL INDEX

White chocolate, 139
Whitman's Sampler, 7
Whole wheat bread, 7
Wise Potato Chips, 10, 27, 149
Wolfing down food, 18

Yodels, 17
York Peppermint Patties, 131

Zero, 131
Zinger, 17

GEOGRAPHICAL INDEX

Lafayette Coney Island (burgers), 51, 56
Monty's Grill (burgers), 51, 56
Nemo's (burgers), 50, 55
Woodbridge Tavern (burgers), 50, 55

Minnesota
Minneapolis
Al's (breakfast), 81
Matin (egg rolls), 72
Minneapolis Technical Institute (best
deal), 75
Rosebud Grocery, 83
Windfield Potter's (all you can eat), 77
St. Paul
Awada (happy hour), 85
Cherokee Sirloin Room, 79

Missouri
Kansas City
Mario's (grinders), 68
St. Louis
Amighetti Bakery, 47–48
Cheshire Inn (all you can eat), 76–77
Crown Candy Kitchen, 62
Cyrano's (top ten), 113–114
Miss Hulling's (cafeteria), 41
Miss Hulling's Creamery (ice cream), 62
Pasta House (all you can eat), 76
Sesame Seed Cookies, 65
Spicer's 5 & 10 (best penny candy), 73

New Jersey
Atlantic City
White House (hoagies), 86
Cherry Hill
Bayard's (unusual chocolate), 70
Big John's (cheesesteaks), 107
South Orange
Town Hall Delicatessen (Sloppy Joe), 67

New York
Brooklyn
Nathan's (hot dogs), 39, 89, 137
Junior's (cheesecake), 30, 102
Buffalo
Anchor Bar (chicken wings), 111
Endicott
Pat Mitchell's (ice cream), 61
Ithaca
Noyes Lodge (Cornell U.), 43
Manhattan
B & H Dairy Luncheonette, 102
Betsy's Place (cookies), 65
Bonté (bakery), 45
Broome Street Bar (burgers), 50, 53
Burger Joint, 29, 50, 53
Carnegie Delicatessen, 102
Chirping Chicken, 72
Dave's Luncheonette (egg cream), 103
David's Cookies, 65
Dubrow's Cafeteria, 41, 103
Empire Diner (burgers), 51, 53, 73
Erotic Baker, 48
Frusen Glädjé Ice Cream Cart, 97
H & H Bagels, 102
Horn & Hardart Automat, 103
J. G. Melon (burgers), 51, 53
Jackson Hole Wyoming (burgers), 51, 53

John's Pizzeria (top ten), 115–116
Jumbo Hot Bagels, 102
Katz's Delicatessen, 31, 39, 103
LaCart Chevalean (horseburgers), 70
Macy's Cellar (rye bread), 102
Manhattan Market (all you can eat), 76
Mary Elizabeth's Cruller Bar, 38
Miss Grimble (cheesecake), 102
Moondance (burgers), 51, 53
Ray's Pizza, 103
Rumbuls (chocolate cake), 74
Sabrett Hot Dog Stands, 39
Second Avenue Delicatessen, 102
South Street Seaport, 83
Supreme Macaroni, 103
Veniero's (bakery), 45
Waverly and Waverly (burgers), 51, 53
Wolf's Delicatessen, 102
Yonah Schimmel (knish bakery), 102
Zabar's (top ten), 102, 118
Southampton
Robert's (ice cream), 61

Ohio
Cincinnati
Graeter's (ice cream), 62
Skyline Chili, 111
Cleveland
West Side Market, 84
Dayton
Pine Club (steak), 78

Pennsylvania
Cuddy
Fatigati's (prime ribs), 82
Philadelphia
Bassett's (ice cream), 61
Comissary (cafeteria), 41
Federal Pretzel Co., 108
Hilary's (ice cream), 61
Jim's Steaks (cheesesteak), 67, 107
Lee's (hoagies), 108
Levis, 40
More than Just Ice Cream, 82
Overbrook (Italian ices), 108 ·
Pat's, King of Steaks (cheesesteak), 107
Philadelphia Soft Pretzel, 108

Tennessee
Nashville
Standard Candy Company, 31

Texas
Austin
Hoffbrau (University of Texas), 43, 78
Dallas
Bishop's Grill (down-home cooking),
106
Chili's (burgers), 51, 55, 101
Dallas Tortilla and Tamale Factory, 100
Dunston's (burgers), 50, 54
Guadalajara (Tex-Mex), 101
Highland Park Cafeteria, 40–41
Highland Park Pharmacy (soda
fountain), 75
Hofbrau (steak), 78
Lightfoot's (burgers), 51, 55
Magic Time Machine (most unusual
theme), 70–71

Rosemarie's (down-home cooking), 106
Snuffer's (burgers), 50, 55, 74
Sonny Bryan's (top ten), 67, 99, 119
Stoneleigh P. (burgers), 51, 55
Tolbert's (chili), 101
Fort Worth
Angelo's (top ten), 99, 119
Kincaid's (burgers), 51, 55
Houston
Alfie's (unusual combination dinner), 70
Bellaire Broiler Burger, 51, 56
Fuddrucker's, 50, 56, 82
Goode Company (barbecue), 99
Hofbrau (steak), 78
James' Restaurant (burgers), 51, 56
Las Cazuelas (Tex-Mex), 101
Luling City Market (barbecue), 99
Neal's (ice cream), 62
Ninfa's (Tex-Mex), 100
Old Bayou Inn (burgers), 51, 56
Otto's (burgers), 51, 56
Roznovsky's (burgers), 50, 56
Shephard Drive Barbecue, 99
Su Casa (Tex-Mex), 101
Texas Bar-B-Que House (best gimmick), 75
Texas Steak Ranch and Saloon (all you can eat), 77
Pasadena
Leisure Boarding House (down-home cooking), 105–106

San Antonio
Los Arcos Cafe (Tex-Mex), 100
Mi Tierra Cafe and Bakery (Tex-Mex), 100
Texas Hot Stuff (Tex-Mex), 100
Sugar Land
Crazy Ed's (chili), 101

Vermont
Burlington
Ben & Jerry's (ice cream), 61

Virginia
Richmond
Bill's Barbecue (best lemonade), 68, 73
Sally Bell's (bakery), 45
Salem
Gwaltney of Smithfield (ham), 31
Virginia Beach
Forbes Candies, 31
Wakefield
Virginia Diner (peanuts), 75

Washington
Seattle
Pike Place Market, 84

Wisconsin
Milwaukee
Solly's (burgers), 57